The Politics of Nursing

Nursing Today is a new series that looks critically yet constructively at the work of nursing and the needs of nurses. Future titles will include *Nursing and Sexuality*, *Stress and Self-care: a Guide for Nurses*, *Holistic Nursing* and *Assertiveness: a Guide for Nurses*.

Nursing Today

The Politics of Nursing

Jane Salvage

Illustrations by Cath Jackson

Foreword by Alison Dunn

Heinemann Nursing

Heinemann Nursing
An imprint of Heinemann Professional Publishing Ltd
Halley Court, Jordan Hill, Oxford OX2 8EJ

OXFORD   LONDON   SINGAPORE
NAIROBI   IBADAN   KINGSTON

First published 1985
Reprinted 1985, 1986, 1987, 1989

© Jane Salvage 1985

ISBN 0 433 29010 2

Typeset by D. P. Media Ltd, Hitchin
Printed and bound in Great Britain by
Biddles Ltd, Guildford and King's Lynn

Contents

He came on to the ward at ten
I was right, he said.
leukaemia
I said he'd got leukaemia, didn't I?

Are the parents here?
Nurse — go and see.
She went, running.
Yes, they're here she said, breathlessly

I'll break it to them, he said
decisively
and broke them

And left the nurse with the pieces.
But she wasn't trained to cope with broken lives
She was only trained
to fetch the stethoscope.

Mary Twomey, district nurse

Foreword

Many nurses are uncomfortable with the word 'politics'. It belongs to a world of which they do not feel, nor want to be, part. Politics is for others. Politics is a deviant activity in which no self-respecting professional should indulge. Politics, moreover, would wither away if only everything could be discussed and decided on a civilised basis.

Jane Salvage's book firmly stamps on these myths, showing just how far 'politics' in its widest possible sense imbues every major problem and preoccupation of nurses today. With a remarkable overview of nursing's historical and sociological context, the book strongly reflects the author's own feminist and socialist beliefs. But far from being a merely polemical treatise, it contains important material which every nurse would find valuable and stimulating.

Above all it is a courageous book. Nursing — profession or occupation — is not renowned for its creative thinking. Nurses are not encouraged to explore their own ideas, to think critically or challenge established ways of doing. It is essentially a docile profession, ready to complain in private but reluctant to speak out in public. Jane has resisted attempts to fall into a conventional nursing mould — and the fruits of her rebellion are contained in this book. The courage this requires should never be underestimated.

I first spotted Jane as one of nursing's shamefully rare

intelligent and articulate politicos, when as a student nurse she attended a Royal College of Nursing annual conference. The editor of *Nursing Mirror* at the time, Mark Allen, was even swifter off the mark than I and Jane was signed up — to my great chagrin — on the rival journal. Her student columns in the *Mirror* were rivetting — a combination of exceptional writing talent and great perception about nurses and nursing. Only later did I learn about the attempt by teachers and managers at her hospital to suppress or at least control what she said. Jane, armed with a Cambridge degree and deep personal beliefs in the power of nursing, withstood the pressure to which thousands before her had succumbed.

When at last Jane and I came to work together, she had become a professional journalist emerging as IPC's top trainee journalist of her year. 'Who would have expected it of a nurse?' people said. She joined *Nursing Times* as a reporter, moving rapidly to news editor and then features editor. Her rigour as a writer and sub-editor was matched only by her wide-ranging grasp of the politics of health care on one hand and the minutiae of nursing's day to day responsibility on the other. Jane set the highest standards for herself and expected all around her to do likewise. This book is the culmination of this heady mixture. Crisply written, well researched, provocative, educational, it cannot fail to stimulate even those who claim not to see what politics has to do with nursing. It has become almost a cliché that nurses must become more political — a catchphrase which few people have so far dared to explore in any depth. This important book reaches far beyond the clichés into the everyday working lives of nurses in Britain.

Alison Dunn
London 1985

Alison Dunn was Editor of *Nursing Times* from 1975 to 1983. She is now Director of Press and Public Relations for the Royal College of Nursing.

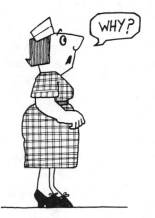

Introduction

Many of the ideas in this book are the product of years of discussion, both formal and informal, in a variety of settings. Primarily my views on and feelings about nursing have been shaped by my own work as a student and staff nurse, but my understanding and analysis have been deepened through participation in the Radical Nurses Group, the Politics of Health Group and several other groups and activities. These discussions are continuing and I hope this book will be seen very much as a contribution to that process rather than as a finished product. My aim is not to state unequivocal conclusions but to encourage debate in areas which have been relatively unexplored or even taboo in nursing.

Because of the way this book came to be written, it is particularly hard to decide to whom I owe the biggest debt of gratitude for giving me the strength and support to finish it, and for helping me to develop the ideas. The Radical Nurses Groups in London, Manchester and Sheffield and also nationwide were the original inspiration for the book — through our desire to spread our ideas to a wider audience, especially to ordinary working nurses. Many individual people contributed much and, at the risk of leaving someone out, I would like to thank them by name, as well as others who supported me in different ways: Angie Cotter, Michelle Davies, Heulwen Evans, Pattie Grutchfield, Caroline

MacKeith, Jan Savage, Eileen Sheehan, Pam Smith, Mary Twomey and Cathy Watson.

I would like to thank Cath Jackson not just for producing the marvellous illustrations, but for doing them with such sensitivity and commitment to nurses and to this project. The book also contains verbatim comments from a number of nurses, mostly anonymous, and I would like to thank them too for their contribution.

I'd like to take this opportunity to explain some aspects of the text. First, gender and grammar. Conventionally, books about nursing refer to nurses throughout as 'she', and to doctors and patients as 'he'. This can be regarded as an accurate generalisation for nurses, since less than one in ten people doing paid nursing work is male. For doctors 'he' is less accurate, since the gender ratio at junior level is roughly half and half — although the medical establishment is thoroughly male-dominated. For patients 'he' is inaccurate since more women than men use the NHS.

In this book I refer to nurses as 'she' where neutrality cannot be avoided, not only because there are more female nurses but because nursing is still predominantly a female culture; in the same spirit I refer to doctors as 'he'. Where it is unavoidable patients are referred to as 'he' for simplicity only.

Secondly I would like to explain my somewhat unorthodox reference system. Since this is intended as a discussion document rather than a scholarly treatise — though I believe my conclusions are justifiable! — I have decided not to scatter the text too liberally with references. Many of the articles and books I mention develop or debate the ideas I raise, rather than confirming the validity or otherwise of what I write. Others indeed contradict my ideas but contain useful or interesting arguments or information. Therefore, primarily in the hope of encouraging the reader to turn to other sources, I have not numbered the references in the text, but have listed them at the end of each chapter or section as 'Further Reading'. Please note that these suggestions may relate to more than one chapter or section, but that for brevity I have included them only where they first appear.

London 1985   Jane Salvage

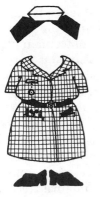

What
is a nurse?

have the images chose

Everyone thinks they know what a nurse is. She is a young woman who wears a distinctive uniform and a crisp white cap and works in a hospital looking after sick people. Everyone, too, thinks they know what a nurse does: she carries out the doctor's orders so that illness can be cured, and she helps the sick person through this painful process with comforts drawn from her reserves of compassion and common sense — mopping the fevered brow here, offering a word of reassurance there.

The image of the nurse also carries warm and tender associations which go back to our earliest intimate experiences. To breastfeed is to nurse, and 'Nurse' was also the name once given to women who were paid to mother middle-class children. This link between the nurse and motherhood, which plays its part in the relationships between nurses and patients, is reinforced by the idea of feeding and nourishing which is implied when we use the word 'nurse' metaphorically, such as in 'nursing a grievance' — nurturing feelings in the very core of our being.

This first experience of being nursed, nourished physically and emotionally by a strong female figure, is almost universal. And although some men, in different societies and at different times, may play a part in caring for children, it is usually women who perform those vital tasks of nurturing.

In Britain today women look after sick children, partners and other ill people, whether in a small family unit or a larger network, while relatively few men do so. Despite the existence of the National Health Service and the replacement of traditional kinds of care with supposed professional expertise, most nursing continues to happen outside institutions, carried out by women with no special training. Hundreds of thousands of people with health problems — chronic diseases, physical disabilities, problems caused by old age or mental handicap — are looked after at home. Sometimes they may be supported by a community nurse or a home help, but the majority depend heavily on relatives and friends, usually women; when those women in turn need care, they generally have to rely on the welfare state.

So although our first notion of the nurse is someone who is paid to care for strangers in an institution, nursing is not the prerogative of the trained nurse, a fact which has important implications for the status and development of the occupation. Indeed, the idea that special training is needed to supplement women's supposedly instinctive caring attributes is relatively new. Even the introduction of formal training in the 19th century had more to do with the needs of the medical profession than with the notion that caring was a skill which should be developed through training. The growth of 'scientific medicine' and its development in hospitals created a need for doctors to have assistants who would do their bidding and keep the place in order. Florence Nightingale's belief that patients needed nursing care, spiritual support and a healthy environment was subsidiary to the doctors' requirements.

The move to ensure that people working as paid nurses should be brought under legal control by entering them on an official register was hotly contested and did not become law until 1919. Most nursing was still done at home by female relatives and neighbours, or sometimes by paid private nurses, and attempts were made to control this activity too. Welfare workers and health visitors told women how to bring up their children, while the increasing faith in medicine eroded the use of traditional methods of healing

Edars away
cantid

and curing — often hitherto a female preserve. Women as healers, carers or midwives were no longer to be trusted to do the right things, yet women were still expected to perform nursing tasks as an instinctive female activity.

Today there are still plenty of people, including nurses themselves, who believe that 'good nurses are born, not made'. A Department of Health recruitment advertisement in the late 1970s declared that 'the best nurses have the essential qualifications before they go to school' — in other words, they don't really need much knowledge or education in acquiring physical or mental skills, but can rely on their innate compassion and common sense. Doing a degree in nursing, an option now offered by a number of universities and polytechnics, is viewed with suspicion and incomprehension by nurses and others. Why on earth, they ask, should a nurse want or need a degree? The trend for schools of nursing to require A-levels from applicants, wrote one typical correspondent to *Nursing Times* in April, 1983, 'detracts substantially from the skills needed for good, basic nursing care'.

The reality, though, while nursing's leaders argue about entrance requirements, is that most people in hospital or outside it are nursed by people with no formal training or

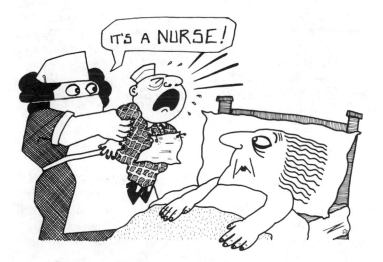

qualification. In most areas of the health service, trained nurses have always been outnumbered by unqualified staff and students. Nursing auxiliaries and assistants (who are not legally entitled to be called 'nurse') have no formal training except, occasionally, an odd day in school, and they make up about a quarter of the NHS nursing workforce. Student and pupil nurses, i.e. those in training for a statutory qualification, add up to another quarter. Some of the trained staff hold senior posts in management and education, so the proportion of trained to untrained nurses actually working with patients is lower than 50:50. In many long-stay hospitals, in particular, the bulk of the nursing work is carried out by untrained staff.

Nursing is not only a matter of helping people overcome physical illness. Psychiatric nurses are concerned with people who are mentally ill, while those working with mentally handicapped people are not really concerned with illness at all, but with people who are permanently disabled. Others, like health visitors, offer a mainly advisory service, while school nurses check the health of schoolchildren. Midwives, who need not be nurses at all, supervise normal childbirth. In short, nursing comprises a huge range of activities carried out by a huge number of people. There are nearly 200 000 trained nurses in the NHS, 78 000 nursing students, and 105 000 auxiliaries and assistants, and innumerable women and men nursing people at home. Making generalisations about such a many-headed monster is a dangerous business. But nurses' own testimony, the history of the occupation and the position it holds in society do come together and illuminate each other through a number of themes which this book will explore.

Women's work

Most nurses are women and it is still regarded as a woman's job, with the possible exception of psychiatry where the image of the male nurse as custodian or attendant is still strong. In the media, nursing has an almost exclusively female image, and the attributes of the ideal nurse are those of the ideal woman. Even today nurses are told that their training is good preparation for being a wife and mother. Unstinting compassion and self-sacrifice are the virtues not only of the angels of mercy but of the perfect woman, though other values may be emphasised according to the needs of society and of men in particular.

Any occupational group dominated by women will be subject to society's value-judgements about supposedly female attributes and capabilities. In nursing, our physical and psychological intimacy with patients and our quasi-domestic duties are closely allied to tasks traditionally regarded as women's 'natural' sphere. In the 19th century this view of nursing as an extension of work inside the home was exploited by middle-class women like Florence Nightingale who were desperate to find a legitimate activity outside it. They won acceptance, on the whole, not by challenging explicitly the medical profession's control of hospital care but by presenting themselves as skilled domestic managers, less likely to be seen as a threat to medical power. Nightingale had no illusions about men's superior abilities or intellect, to judge by her early essay *Cassandra*, but she nevertheless decided to subordinate her nurses to the doctors. This tactic helped to establish nursing in hospitals, and its legacy for good or ill remains with us.

The housekeeping emphasis of the early trail-blazers was partly a result of Nightingale's belief in a clean and healthy environment for the sick. But they also turned their backs on the centuries of work done by female healers, who did not make the now popular distinction between cure and care. Instead, the early matrons adopted a subservient position to the new men of science, though they held sway in their own domestic empires.

Although the link with traditional female work was partly a strategy adopted by the matrons to win acceptance, they did not necessarily think household duties were low in status. They were middle and upper-class women who brought to the hospital the skills described in books like *Mrs. Beeton's Household Management*. These skills were numerous and varied and involved directing a staff of servants; the

Ms Beeken

Victorian patriarch did not interfere (although he established the parameters). The matrons built themselves a formidable power base by creating a similar sphere of influence in major hospitals. They did not challenge male authority and they exerted tight control over the working-class women who did much of the basic work. Today, though, nursing is held in low esteem because of its link with domestic labour. Nearly one in 20 employed women has a nursing job, but as a career choice it faces stiff competition. The wider opportunities brought by better education for women and the opening up of old male strongholds have made nursing less appealing, and many potential nurses are put off by its old-fashioned and stuffy image.

Many nurses do not like to acknowledge the domestic link. Some point to the number of male nurses as proof of its higher status, though the upward mobility of men in nursing suggests that many have little regard for 'basic' nursing and its poor pay and conditions. The ratio of men to women in nursing averages one to 8·5, but the higher you go in the career ladder, the greater the concentration of men. There is one male auxiliary to every 19 women, but the ratio in senior posts is one to one. Men who move up, of course, gradually shake off the stigma of doing women's work — as they move away from the actual practice of nursing and into management and education.

Men in nursing reject the idea of it being close to domestic work, and so do nursing leaders in the professional organisations and statutory bodies. They do not pay much attention to low pay and poor conditions at the bottom of the scale, or to the fact that nurses are badly treated because they are women, whose job is undervalued and whose pay is seen merely as pin money. Public sector unions like COHSE and NUPE are beginning to use these arguments under pressure from their women members who are a numerical majority, but on the whole the self-styled progressives, trying to establish nursing as a profession, tend to undervalue the work of women as carers in the family and managers of the household. They see its low social status, but they accept the status quo and fail to insist that society should rethink its values.

Junior nurses, too, tend to undervalue the importance of caring and of the 'basic' nursing tasks of bed bathing, pressure area care or simple conversation; they say it is not 'real nursing'. As these jobs can be and often are performed by untrained auxiliaries, the students and juniors see their professional status vested in more technological tasks, and distance themselves from the work which has a demeaning link with domesticity. 'Proper nursing' is now being seen as the more 'scientific' jobs like giving injections, minding machines, and performing other tasks routinely done by doctors (who are only too pleased to pass on their own low-status work). This low value ascribed to 'basic nursing' by nurses themselves both reflects and reinforces society's prejudices.

However, the way our health care system divides the work of looking after sick and handicapped people appears to be lagging behind the gradually changing perceptions of women's role and status in society as a whole. The curing function is regarded as the province of doctors, usually men, and caring is the province of nurses, usually women — a gender division of labour which reflects the traditional gender stereotyping of skills and qualities. Decisive behaviour, rational thinking and competitiveness are seen as masculine attributes, while irrationality, docility and sacrificing personal needs are feminine attributes. People who deviate from these types are labelled disapprovingly; so assertive women are 'aggressive' and compassionate men are 'effeminate', though their behaviour would be regarded as natural in the opposite sex. This tyranny is reflected in general health care: doctors, the active curers, are seen as scientists — logical thinkers who can be relied on to make tough decisions based on hard fact — while passive nurses give tender loving care. In reality, of course, the work does not divide neatly in that way, but we have what amounts to a silent conspiracy to preserve the myth.

This gender division of health care labour has had far-reaching consequences for nurses. Like other women workers, nurses have low pay and low status and lack political muscle, yet their work underpins the supposed miracle cures of doctors — who enjoy massive salaries, immense social status and a monopoly control of their profession. Despite the complementary nature of medicine and nursing work, doctors have mostly failed to support nurses in pay struggles or any other struggle; the politically stronger group has failed to support the weaker.

The status of an occupation is often measured by its pay and conditions, and medicine is supposed *per se* to be more valuable and difficult than nursing, despite the 'you nurses are wonderful' compliments. The two jobs are viewed in a hierarchical relationship, and even highly qualified nurses are still seen as failed doctors, for example by Polly Toynbee writing in *World Medicine*, March 1983. The doctor is always a personality and his foibles or even rudeness are indulged almost as the hallmarks of his superiority, whereas nurses have little individuality and are interchangeable. Curing is held to require years of education, while caring is held to be instinctive.

Nurses know, though they often lack the confidence to assert it, that caring is difficult. Some go further and reject the care/cure division altogether. The more we learn about health, the more we are realising that it depends on many factors, emotional, physical, environmental and so on. Who can say with certainty why one person recovers from a disease and another does not? Who can say whether it is the 'cure' — the operation, perhaps — or the postoperative 'care' and rehabilitation which is more important in recovery? Besides, the very notion of cure is irrelevant to many handicapped and long-term sick people using the NHS, to whom modern medicine, unlike modern nursing, has little to offer.

Health services in the West tend to divide the work along these gender lines. But a sexual division of labour is also taking place inside nursing. In the early days women entered general nursing while men opted for psychiatry and mental handicap, but now the general field is coming to be dominated by men, not in numbers but in leadership. For example, the Royal College of Nursing excluded men until 1960 but now has a male general secretary, male full-time officials and many male activists. In education the top posts are occupied by a disproportionate number of men, and some women are already expressing concern at the lack of female role models.

On the whole, though, this has been seen as progress. More men in nursing, it is claimed, will raise its status, and some male nurses say the growing political awareness of nurses is their doing. They supposedly bring managerial know-how, industrial relations expertise and willingness to fight for their rights, while their very presence is seen as a challenge to medical domination. Some nurses — male and female — argue that men are more likely to be heeded in the multidisciplinary, mainly male teams which manage the health service, and moreover most of the new general manager jobs are going to men. In other words, the men will sort the women out, and they are taking to this with alacrity, as many a nursing conference, statutory body or union hierarchy demonstrates.

One view suggests that the old domination of female nurses by women of a higher class, the matrons, is being replaced with the domination of women by male nurses. Not only are the men coming to outnumber women in senior posts, but the emphasis on nursing as a series of scientific, technical and sub-medical tasks indicates a belief in masculine rather than feminine values (science being mistakenly thought of as masculine, rational and value-free). This is echoed in the pseudo-industrial style of nursing management, with its emphasis on manpower (*sic*) planning, cost-effectiveness, problem-solving and decision-making.

Male nurses of course find such criticisms upsetting, and defend themselves with talk of discrimination. But what's sauce for the goose may not be sauce for the gander if your goose is about to be cooked! Most female nurses respect the courage of men who fight prejudice to work in a traditionally female job, but that does not in itself allay the fears aroused by the disproportionate number of men in top posts, because those men are likely to have different priorities from the women. As Austin pointed out in *Nursing Times* in 1977, 'for most male nurses a nursing career denotes a career in a service occupation, whereas for most female nurses a nursing career means a lifetime of service.'

As in nearly all other jobs it is easier for men to get to the top. The usually unmarried women who provided nursing's leadership in the past failed miserably to make provision for women with family commitments to pursue their occupations and develop their talents. The pressure of doing two jobs — one paid, in the hospital or clinic, and one unpaid, in the home — still deters many women from seeking promotion or doing more specialised work. In 1977 there were almost as many part-time nursing staff as full-timers (excluding students), but few workplaces provide crèches, payment for childminders, job-sharing or other schemes to help women who work and care for children. The part-timers are effectively penalised for having children, and the way is left open for the men to move upwards. Instead of fighting for a re-evaluation of the work traditionally done by women, many of the men are trying to move away from it, into education and administration, as fast as they can.

The nurse's role in health care

Many people have tried to define the role of the nurse in health care, but no one definition can encompass all the activities involved, even if it is restricted to the work of people holding statutory nursing qualifications. Nurses work in a variety of fields, from the largely preventive, advisory work of health visitors to the highly technical, curatively oriented field of intensive care — as different as chalk and cheese. The tasks done by any single nurse in one shift usually include complex and delicate discussion with a patient, technical procedures demanding considerable manual dexterity, and unskilled jobs like emptying bedpans. As Florence Nightingale said in her *Notes on Nursing* in 1860, 'I use the word nursing for want of a better.'

It is difficult, then, to devise a definition of nursing which is not so broad as to be almost meaningless. Yet many of the deep disagreements among nurses, and between them and other workers, are concerned with interpreting the proper

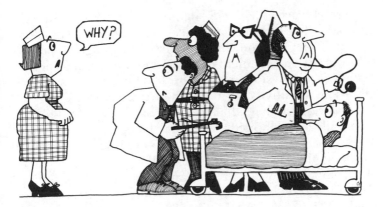

role of the student, manager and so on. Are health visitors, for example, doing work which should be done by social workers? Is making beds a sensible use of the time of a qualified nurse? Should nursing auxiliaries be encouraged to check blood pressure and should students give out drugs? There are no easy answers, but such questions are relevant even to those who may dislike rigid definition of roles, since they are a major preoccupation in nursing today.

Trying to work out what the role of the nurse is and could be is not just an academic exercise. It has occupied many minds and produced some fatuous as well as some enlightening conclusions, and should not be used as an excuse to berate nurses who fail or refuse to conform to a set of rigid guidelines. But without a working definition of some kind, we lack a starting point. A sensible appraisal of what the nurse does is needed as a springboard to help us decide what nursing work should aim to be doing — and what its priorities should be. The need for nurses to set their goals has never been as urgent as it is today, when they are under pressure from all sides — from doctors, cost-conscious health authorities, and increasingly articulate and demanding users of the NHS.

Most people, including nurses, would define their job as looking after sick people, with the aim of reducing their suffering and nursing them back to health. But the growing complexity of modern health care, and the needs of the people who use the NHS, demand a more sophisticated approach. The technical advances of medicine and its capacity to prolong life, the changing needs of an ageing population and the development of specialties and occupations like dietetics and physiotherapy point to a need for greater flexibility and sensitivity on the part of the 'carers'.

A basic question is what we mean by illness. Mentally and physically handicapped people may have mental or physical illnesses caused by their disabilities, but are they, strictly speaking, ill? They cannot be 'cured' and modern medicine often has little to offer them, and their disability is not a temporary state but a lifelong problem. They do not usually need nursing in the traditional sense of nurturing them through a period of sickness, but they do need expert help to encourage them to make the most of the abilities they have and to develop new ones. Old people are another group who are increasingly occupying the attention of health workers, but old age should not be regarded as a disease, although longer life expectancy means people are surviving to wrestle with the difficulties caused by minds and bodies which are simply wearing out. The support they need is not necessarily in being looked after, but in learning how to cope with such problems as memory lapses, decreasing mobility or incontinence, and finding out what help they can get from state and voluntary agencies for equipment, services and so on.

Changing attitudes to mental illness are also tending to emphasise growth and self-help, with the nurse's role moving away from that of custodian to one of therapist, offering the patient or client support and encouragement to be independent. The care of physical illness, too, has swung away from keeping patients in bed for weeks towards much more active forms of recuperation. Nursing, though, is taking a long time to adapt to such changes. Nurses still tend to dress the elderly man or lift the stroke patient to her chair rather than teach them how to do it themselves, even though their chances of returning to an active life will be improved by support from people who can develop their practical skills, rather than treat them like helpless children.

Even here, though, generalisations are crude. Part of the

nurse's skill is learning to recognise when to lend a helping hand and when to forbear, for there are always times when even the most determined person needs to have their load shared or removed. Thus the nurse needs psychological as well as physical expertise, and the opportunity to know her patients as people and to respect their right to decide what they need.

Recent attempts to define the nurse's role have taken all this into account, though textbook definitions are of course a long way from what is practised in homes and hospitals. One of the most useful starting points, and probably the most often quoted, was formulated by the American nurse Virginia Henderson: 'The unique function of the nurse is to assist the individual, sick or well, in the performance of those activities contributing to health or its recovery (or to peaceful death) that he would perform unaided if he had the necessary strength, will or knowledge. And to do this in such a way as to help him gain independence as rapidly as possible.' (Quoted in *Basic Principles of Nursing Care*, p. 4, published by the International Council of Nurses, Geneva, 1969.)

In the UK, the committee on nursing which produced the Briggs report in 1972, a major and comprehensive survey of modern nursing, reached a conclusion about the nurse's role which linked it more directly to the environment in which she works. Her central role is always, it said, 'to ensure the care and comfort of the person being nursed, to maintain oversight and co-ordination of that care and to integrate the whole — both preventive and curative — into an appropriate social context.' But this rather static view lacks Henderson's emphasis on the nurse as a force in the dynamic, continuing process towards health and independence, and fails to assign any precise meaning to the 'appropriate social context'.

More recently some of the constraints under which nurses work have been highlighted by the Royal College of Nursing in its consideration of the role of the nurse. In its report *Standards of Nursing Care* (1980), it looked at the nurse as overseer and coordinator of all the work concerned with patient care. Although it believes the nurse is responsible for ensuring that patients receive whatever they need in treatment, care or services, the RCN acknowledges that the nurse has no formal control over any other staff group or service, either in the hospital or the community. Such a broad view of the nurse's place in health care is treading dangerously close to sensitive medical toes, and the RCN fails to tackle this explicitly. The lid will not be kept on it for ever, though, and doctors are showing great unease at the challenge to their supremacy which is implied in the growing mood of independence among nurses. Situations where the nurse's professional judgement conflicts with the doctor's — and where the nurse is prepared to voice disagreement — are becoming more common by the month, and have already made headline news in incidents like that at Wexham Park Hospital in Slough, where the psychiatric unit's senior nurse was dismissed after refusing to administer, without the patient's consent, an injection ordered by a doctor.

The reaction of Wexham Park's psychiatrist, Peter Maddocks, to this nursing challenge is probably fairly typical of many doctors, and shows the hostility nurses will face if they attempt to define and establish any role in isolation from other disciplines. The medical profession in particular has enormous power to block any change. Writing in *The Consultant* in December 1982, Dr Maddocks put forward his own sarcastic interpretation of how nurses saw their role: 'Nursing is a profession. Nurses are professionals. Professionals are independent and of independent judgement. A nurse is as likely to be right in her opinion about a patient as any other professional. Nursing care is provided continuously for in-patients. A nurse spends longer with a patient than anyone else, and therefore has more observation on which to base her opinion. Therefore a nurse's opinion on a patient is more likely to be correct than anyone else's.'

His article, and the journal's editorial, had no doubts about how to deal with such heretical and presumptious attitudes on the part of nurses; both were determined to see the developments in nursing purely as a means of replacing one form of authority over the patient with another. 'Consultants must be in charge and be seen to be in charge,' it declared. 'Authority should be delegated sparingly, preferably to other consultants ... challenges to consultant authority must be dealt with sympathetically but firmly ... the alternative is the risk of anarchy.'

What the doctors are refusing to acknowledge, and what is also highlighted by the RCN, is a growing tension within nursing about the division between the 'caring' and 'curing' aspects of the work. 'Nursing is increasingly becoming an extension of the doctor's diagnostic and curative role,' the college notes; the tasks increasingly being undertaken by nurses, such as assessing patients in the community or giving intravenous chemotherapy, used to be regarded as medical tasks. The dilemma about where and how the nurse should concentrate her activity is becoming more acute. Taking on these specialist tasks could be a step forward to independence from medical domination — but it could just be making life easier for the doctors by taking on their simpler routine work, which will become routine for nurses too once the thrill of innovation has gone.

The RCN sees dangers in this increasing specialisation. The value and strength of nursing, it says, lies in its 'adaptive and generalist nature', in the nurse's ability to represent specialists like doctors and physiotherapists in their absence and to adapt her work accordingly. The attributes of continuity and adaptability are likely to become more important with the fragmentation of patient care through specialisation, for each patient in hospital is seen by a bewildering variety of people, each with a different function, and only the nursing service provides 24-hour continuity. Specialist roles such as behaviour therapist or stoma therapist offer advantages to patient and nurse, says the college, but 'a careful balance between generalist and specialist nursing roles needs to be maintained.'

This theory about nursing as 'continuous and adaptive' shows the difficulty of solving the old arguments about 'non-nursing duties', or perhaps sidesteps them. Nurses often complain that they have to do tasks which could and should be done by other workers, and that doing these so-called non-nursing duties takes up the time they could otherwise spend on the job they have been trained to do. Paperwork and menial jobs like washing up or serving tea are often seen in this light, and cuts in NHS funding have increased the pressure on nurses to do such jobs in the absence of other staff — clerical or domestic, for example. Nurses are often left feeling that they carry the can when times are difficult and staff is short. As the only service in constant contact with patients, they have little choice but to do the work (a view also held by many nurses when other staff go on strike). This 'adaptive' role therefore needs to be handled with care if it is not simply to be used as an excuse for exploitation.

On the other hand, nurses complain about the fragmentation which accompanies a strict insistence on demarcation between the jobs of different workers. Giving out meals has been regarded by some nurses from Nightingale onwards as an important nursing task, but many hospitals now have dietitians to work out patients' menus and domestics to serve them. Does this mean nurses have more time for 'real nursing', or does it detract from their overview of each patient's needs and progress, of which nutrition is an important part?

Such arguments often come to the fore during industrial action. Even nurses who belong to trade unions and support such action often feel obliged to stay at work and look after the patients, and the unions make some effort to acknowledge their difficult position — though arrangements for 'emergency cover' are often viewed with scepticism since low staffing levels mean many wards do no better in 'normal' circumstances. Nurses are often under strong pressure from management to do jobs normally undertaken by clerical staff, domestics, orderlies or porters, and those nurses who refuse on principle have no precise job description by which to exempt themselves. Arguing that they do not do certain jobs through 'custom and practice' is difficult, too, when staffing fluctuates within nursing and among other workers from one shift to another.

The exclusion of 'non-nursing duties' from the nurse's role has other implications. Some nurses are using it as part of their strategy to establish nursing as a profession; just as real professionals like doctors and lawyers do not do mundane tasks like making beds or pushing trolleys, neither, they argue, should trained nurses. They do not heed the more radical view that a just and civilised society might try to share out the menial work, so the nursing auxiliary as well as the ward sister could have her share of satisfying and interesting work, and would be regarded as making a valuable contribution too.

An excessively rigid definition of the nurse's role, then, may not be the best option. Yet nurses' sense of responsibility and compassion has often been exploited, and at a time when the NHS is desperately short of resources, it is vital that they do not allow themselves to be used to paper over the cracks. Professional jealousies and demarcation disputes thrive when people are feeling threatened and defensive, and nursing should avoid those traps. As a bridge between all groups of staff, nurses are in a unique position to be a positive force, and for our sakes as well as the patients' we must be clear about our aims and priorities.

Further Reading

Austin R. (1977). Sex and Gender in the Future of Nursing. *Nursing Times*, Occasional Papers; August 25 and September 1.

Carpenter M. (1977). The New Managerialism and Professionalism in Nursing. In *Health Care and the Division of Labour* (Stacey M., ed.) London: Croom Helm.

Chamberlain M. (1981). *Old Wives' Tales*. London: Virago.

Ehrenreich D., English B. (1974). *Witches, Midwives and Nurses: A History of Women Healers*. Glass Mountain pamphlet No. 1. London: Compendium.

Nightingale F. (1979). *Cassandra — an Essay*. New York: Feminist Press. (To be published by Virago in the UK in 1986.)

Nightingale F. (1980). *Notes on Nursing*. Edinburgh: Churchill Livingstone.

Report of the Committee on Nursing (Briggs Report; 1972). London: HMSO. See Chapter II, *Nurses and Midwives and the Public: Image and Realities*.

Standards of Nursing Care (an RCN discussion document; 1980). London: Royal College of Nursing.

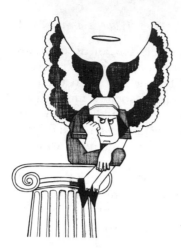

2

Images
and reality

The nurse in uniform is instantly recognisable, and even very small children draw pictures of Nurse in a white cap and apron. Uniforms themselves exert a kind of fascination and it's not surprising that the combination of uniformed women, high drama and illness and death should have made the nurse such a popular figure in the media.

Films, novels, newspapers, documentaries, soap operas, cartoons, recruitment advertising and even get well cards all bombard us with images of the nurse. And despite the variety of sources, and the many different kinds of nurses and nursing work, these images are remarkably consistent. They focus not on what the nurse does but on the way she is supposed to look — female, uniformed, young, white. She is seen not as a skilled worker who tries to do a difficult and complex job, but as a selfless ministering angel whose devotion to the doctor and whose tireless efficiency as his handmaiden enable him, the true professional, to do his job while she soothes the patient's fevered brow.

There are some exceptions, of course; moreover the image of the nurse could more accurately be described as a cluster of stereotypes, a complex series of interconnected images. All have one thing in common, though — the nurse is female. But before looking at where these images come from and how far they reflect nursing as it really is, we need to be convinced that they are important. After all, *Carry On Nurse* and doctor–nurse romances are only fiction, so do they matter? Is there anything wrong with a bit of escapism?

There is much evidence that, like it or not, we are all strongly influenced by the media. Many of us like to be sceptical about advertising — but it works, otherwise companies would not spend millions of pounds on it. We like to find the best value for money, but clever promotion can persuade us to try something new and perhaps more expensive, and it is becoming so sophisticated that some ads are virtually in code, relying on our barely conscious recognition of previous ads rather than a description of the product's merits.

Neither is the power of media images confined to advertising, which is at least explicit in its attempts to influence people. Films and TV provide all sorts of images on which we model ourselves, and even if we consciously reject what is being portrayed, we may subconsciously absorb it and try to conform to it. The women's movement has argued that the way women are depicted on magazine covers and in films is not only unrealistic, but puts pressure on women to try and look like cover girls, and makes them feel inadequate if they don't succeed.

The images around us which provide some of the models by which we judge ourselves are often linked to the patterns of behaviour expected of us all, male and female, from early childhood. Little girls who are given dolls to play with are probably more likely to grow up conscious of their nurturing, mothering role as women, while little boys who've played with guns may be more likely to make their way in the world through aggression. There are of course biological differences between the sexes, but unfortunately these have been used to justify imposing set patterns of 'acceptable' behaviour on men and women, and set ways of expressing ourselves, which may not coincide with our own individual desires, needs or capabilities.

The media images are not something 'out there' or outside ourselves, but act like those early childhood pressures to make us conform to accepted patterns by supporting society's ways of thinking about people — ways of thinking which have tended to uphold the domination of women by men in the public and social sphere. Doctor–nurse relationships in romantic novels are not so far removed from the games when boys are doctors, providing the knowledge and giving the orders, and girls are nurses, providing the compassion and taking the orders.

The images of nurses hardly ever depict men, even though 10% of nurses are male. They are almost exclusively female and generally reflect stereotyped views of women as seen through male eyes — as mothers or sexual partners. Even the *Sun*'s angels and the Hattie Jacques power-mad spinsters are images influenced by the stereotypes, for they are shown to be odd or remarkable because they have rejected the 'natural' destiny of women to be men's mates and mothers to their children.

Angels, battleaxes and sex symbols are the three groups into which most of the images fall. Angels appear so often that in Fleet Street the word is used synonymously with nurses. Innocent, unselfish, utterly dedicated to caring for the sick, they always put service before self; everyone agrees they have been exploited and should be protected, but no-one suggests that they should take their destiny into their own hands. Their submissive nature can perhaps be traced back to one of nursing's roots, the religious orders which provided much of the early institutionalised care. Even the title 'sister' harks back to the convent, as do the chaste white uniforms and starched caps — some hospitals still provide caps which look very like nuns' veils.

Nurses themselves have helped to create this image and have also tried to turn it to their own advantage. Nightingale may not have liked being the Lady with the Lamp but the public adulation of her as a ministering angel gave an essential boost to her efforts to establish a nursing service. Other 19th century nursing reformers used an idealised angelic image alongside gross caricatures of pauper nurses to show the attributes of the 'new nurse' and to persuade Victorian parents that nursing was a seemly occupation for their daughters.

Today, the vocational qualities vested in the angel figure are often emphasised to nursing students as their suggested professional goal. Dedication and service to others are put alongside patience, compliance, and a refusal to be ruffled or to show feelings of anger or hurt. The 'good nurse' does not complain but accepts with grace and composure everything thrown at her, and self-sacrifice is seen as a virtue — to the point where nurses are even heard to argue that raising wages would attract the wrong kind of people into nursing, and that low pay ensures getting 'the right kind of girl' who works not for money but for altruism.

The implication is that any nurse who does show her feelings, who speaks up and asks questions when confused, who does not automatically accept what her seniors tell her but wants evidence to be able to reach her own conclusions, is not an angel but a trouble-maker, unsuitable and not a good nurse. A reasonable refusal to be exploited, to take on two people's work or to take the blame for others' mistakes is not angelic. The innate conservatism of the angel is so strong that many nurses cannot believe that the aim of helping others is more readily achieved through energy and intelligence rather than dumb acquiescence.

The angel label is also an easy way for the public to show their gratitude for the work nurses do. Many patients are genuinely grateful and admiring: 'I wouldn't do your job for a million pounds.' Governments, too, use the same kind of language. Many nurses like this image of themselves, and fail to see that it has become a substitute for positive action to improve their pay and conditions. Moreover, the constant repetition of the praise is stale and ultimately devalues the virtues it is supposed to prize. If all nurses are angels simply because they are nurses, not because they do the job especially well, it's an empty compliment.

Another problem with the angels is that they tend, unless rescued by marriage, to age into battleaxes. The dedication which is depicted so charmingly in the soft young nurse turns into fanaticism in the middle-aged spinster, shown in the image of the fierce ward sister who insists on having the beds in a straight line and makes the junior nurses cry. Like the angel images, these dragons are a nurse version of a stereotype often applied to women in general — old maids who, failing to marry and have children as women 'should', turn sour and vent their frustrations in petty tyranny. These sisters and matrons are never shown organising the ward work or using their clinical skills; instead, they sweep through the ward while everyone stands to attention, like Hattie Jacques in *Carry On Doctor*, or become evil manipulators like Big Nurse in Kesey's *One flew over the cuckoo's nest*, who gets her revenge on men by terrorising her patients.

Again the precursors of these stereotypes can partly be found in nursing's history. The middle-class women who were Miss Nightingale's matrons were mostly single and there is still a high proportion of single women in senior posts. Ward sisters at teaching hospitals tend to be single and often live in hospital accommodation and socialise in female cliques. At one time it was assumed that a nurse would cut short her training if she married. Today, though, many nurses are married; probably an overwhelming majority of the part-timers who comprise 40% of the nursing workforce are married, as well as many of the full-timers.

The angel and the dragon are old favourites, but in the last 20 years they have been joined by a third stereotype which has become the most popular of all — the nurse as sex symbol. Barbara Windsor in the *Carry On* films is perhaps the best known (and her sexy nurse is interchangeable with all the other dumb blonde characters she portrays), but there are many other examples of the feather-brained female who wears black stockings and whose main interest is flirting with the houseman. Newspapers love pin-ups of nurses in bikinis, captioned 'What the doctor ordered . . .', and the busty nurse is a favourite subject of seaside joke postcards, get well cards and even, one year, the trade union COHSE's Christmas card. Just a bit of fun? These images are the more acceptable end of a spectrum extending to pornographic films which have nurses as the focus of male erotic interest. *Naughty night nurses* and similarly titled films are often to be seen in the cinema clubs of Soho.

Sex-symbol nurses were rarely found before World War II. Beatrice and Philip Kalisch, two American nurses who have extensively studied the public image of the nurse, argue that their appearance coincides with the growth of the women's movement. Rampant commercialism has found that sex is a good selling point for anything from chocolate to cars, but the obsessive linking of women and sexuality, as defined by men and as governed by male desires, has other implications. It might be a defensive masculine response to women taking control of their own lives; it might be a way of insisting on women's subordination and, therefore, their lack of suitability to mount a serious challenge to the male preserves of work and public affairs.

Men suffer from this stereotyping too. The lack of images of men in nursing in the media — although the TV series *Angels* has tried to redress the balance and has had a number of male nurse characters — means people are often surprised to find men working as nurses. A large number of them work in psychiatry and mental handicap, which are rarely depicted anyway, but there are also many men in general nursing, with one male to every five female registered nurses. The failure of the images to reflect reality combines with the belief that nursing is women's work to form the idea — shared by many female nurses — that there is something funny and effeminate about men who choose to do nursing.

From there it is an easy leap to the assumption that all male nurses are homosexual, a label which causes problems for many men going into nursing, whatever their sexual orientation or their choice about making it public. Instead of being supported for their courageous decision to defy the stereotypes and do a job they think is worthwhile, they are labelled as gay and, by implication, not proper men, for society cannot yet cope with the idea that 'real' men can be caring, gentle and compassionate. Nor can it cope with the idea that male homosexuality and 'female' characteristics are not synonymous.

Interestingly, there does appear to be a higher proportion of gay men in nursing than in the male population at large, though of course there are no figures to prove it. It might be that male nurses, having decided to enter a predominantly female occupation, feel more able to be open about their sexual preferences. Perhaps more gay men are attracted to nursing because they expect to meet other gays and find the support and friendship they need. Or perhaps they are attracted to it because it does not seem to demand the macho attributes of stereotypical masculinity. In any case it has nothing to do with their abilities as nurses. Many nurses are lesbian, but lesbianism is not even seen as an issue in nursing, unlike male homosexuality. Perhaps, like Queen Victoria, other nurses choose to believe that it doesn't exist.

How real are the images?

These images are all a distortion of reality. Not only do they fail to reflect the daily concerns and problems of the people who nurse, but they belittle nurses by describing them in stereotyped ways. They only tell part of the story, remaining silent about the fact that many nurses are male; that much nursing takes place outside hospital surgical wards and casualty departments; that many nurses are West Indian, Asian or black British citizens; and that nursing is more than passing scalpels to the doctor, taking temperatures and wiping bottoms.

Most of all, the images sanitise nursing and deny the real hardship and stress of the work. Dealing with the physical and mental needs of numerous patients on a single shift, at a time when most wards are understaffed and the length of stay in hospital is going down, is physically and mentally shattering for the nurse. At the best of times it is a demanding job, and in current circumstances the nurse's ability to cope with those demands is eroded by her knowledge that she cannot do the job as well as she would like to. But what does she feel, confronted by the images of hospitals where the nurses have time to chat up doctors and run errands for them? Perhaps she comes to feel that it is somehow her fault if the job seems more like drudgery than romance.

The myths also give a false impression of what health care

is all about. The stereotype nurse is likely to work in a hospital ward caring for surgical patients or others with diagnosed diseases from which they will soon recover, but the NHS actually deals with many other problems. Over half its beds are occupied by people with long-term problems caused by old age, mental or physical handicap or mental illness. In romantic novels and comedy films, however, doctors cure diseases, nurses clear up the mess and hold the patient's hand, the patient goes home well, and nurse and doctor celebrate by getting married.

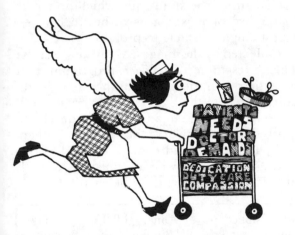

In reality the doctor often does not know what the disease is, or may be unable to do more than alleviate the symptoms. Medicine can do nothing about the factors which cause so much illness today — such as bad housing, unbalanced diets, unsafe conditions at work, accidents, addictions, or stress. Hospital stay for many people, like the 'revolving door' patients in psychiatric hospitals, does not produce cures, but only patches up the damage sufficiently to enable the ill person to go home — and face the same risks all over again.

Nurses are rarely shown working in the community, except for the occasional motherly district nurse on her bike. In fact about one nurse in 10 works outside hospital, doing such diverse jobs as supporting families with a mentally handicapped child, checking schoolchildren's eyesight, helping women look after their babies or counselling people with psychiatric problems. In hospital, the work is equally varied, and even on the surgical ward or theatre beloved by scriptwriters, its scope is enormous.

All this may seem obvious but it is important because it gives people a false picture of what nurses are like and what they do. People accustomed to seeing the nurse in the role of doctor's handmaiden will tend to treat her that way when they become patients, and they may not realise that good nursing care is as vital as medical expertise. They will look to the doctor, not the nurse, for advice and authoritative information, a reinforcement of the status quo which preserves the doctors' dominance of most forms of health care — possibly the biggest single obstacle to progress.

Nurses, too, are affected by the images. Many new recruits expect hospital life to resemble a *Dr Kildare* programme and the effort of readjusting their ideas to what they actually do find (called 'reality shock' in the USA) can be very painful. Even if they themselves manage to adjust and to develop a more realistic attitude to their work, they find that others refuse to accept it. If you are told enough times that you should act as surrogate mother, wife and mistress to both doctors and patients, you might end up believing it.

'(The consultant) smiled up at Anna. "I'll lend you my favourite staff nurse for today. . . ." But Paul Keslar, thoughtfully reading through some of the notes, didn't look up at once. When he did, he said briefly, "I'd better get started then, Sir. We're late enough as it is." Then noticing that Anna was holding open the door for him, he walked purposefully through into the corridor and stood waiting. . . .

Anna worked beside him . . . anticipating his request for instruments or dressings, listening while he made his decisions, firmly and without hesitation, and now she found her respect for him growing hourly . . . In answer to the surgeon's "Goodnight, Staff . . ." she said quietly, still with the smile which was a natural part of her image, "Goodnight, Sir." '

From *The Doctor's Decision*, by Elizabeth Petty, Mills & Boon, London, 1981.

'There were many times when I loved our patients, for they were mostly honest, goodhearted working men and women, and the way in which an imperfect system worked against them always receiving what they deserved, as well as against us giving it, made me angry. But what they did to make me sometimes hate them was to bring their stereotypes of nurses into hospital with them. To some men, the ideal nurse seemed to be Barbara Windsor in a *Carry On* film. Pert, pretty, always good for a naughty giggle, but at the same time chaste little servants without too many brains. The women were more apt to play up the "blessed Virgin" aspect, sometimes almost extolling us as saints minus our haloes. Yet here we are talking of intelligent women, often with two or three A-levels, who are trained to perform technical tasks, and must also have a large capacity for understanding human nature to do their job well.'

Student nurse

In nursing there is plenty of evidence of the way nurses' ideas have been shaped by the stereotypes. Conforming to them may be more comfortable than seeking a more challenging and thoughtful definition of the job, and hiding behind them may help to avoid the problems and the pain of relating to patients and clients as equals and as adults. Nursing leaders, and ironically this is particularly true of those who like to describe nursing as a 'profession', are not immune. The RCN fought a recent pay campaign using posters of nurses with wings and haloes. Nurses who are civil servants have tried to recruit new applicants with literature showing a little girl cuddling a teddy bear.

So look out for the way nurses are portrayed in the media. Next time you see a poster or a hospital film, watch out for the nurses hovering attentively in the background or flaunting their sexual charms. Is this really how you see yourself, and how you want others to see you?

Changing media stereotypes may seem like an uphill task, but some nurses have already found ways to challenge images which they find untruthful or offensive. Feminists have successfully drawn attention to the exploitation of women through pornography, and nurses are learning to use the media to similar positive effect. Complaining to advertisers, journalists or TV producers is one direct and surprisingly effective method. The Advertising Standards Authority does not have a particularly good record on sexism, and approaches to the publications or companies themselves appear to be more constructive; most will publish or answer a complaint letter, while a local newspaper or hospital newsletter may take up the issue as a news story. Nurses in the USA and a few in the UK have started to form 'mediawatch' groups to monitor the representation of nurses and to protest at unacceptable stereotypes. In the USA in 1981 a *Playboy* plan to feature nurses was dropped after telephone, letter and telegram complaints from the Chicago Nurses Association and others (although a similar feature was published in 1983, demonstrating the need for constant vigilance and stronger action).

In the UK much of this kind of activity has been focussed around and generated by the Public Image of Nursing Campaign (PINC). A national conference held in 1983 to discuss PINC's central issues and future strategies gave rise to extensive publicity, including TV and radio interviews enabling nurses to put their case. The effects of such campaigning are impossible to quantify, but at the very least it helped nurses to clarify some ideas and to be more alert to how they themselves might have contributed to a negative image of nursing. The trade unions and professional bodies have also become more sensitive to the issue and are looking at their own role more closely.

Perhaps most importantly, though, nurses have begun to talk to each other much more. Encouraged by more open attitudes in training and a greater sense of the need to discuss and explore what is going on, people are more ready to question others; a stereotypical or belittling comment about nurses, whether it comes from a doctor, a nurse or anyone else, is perhaps less likely today to pass without comment.

Dress uniform

Uniform is an important component of the nurse's public image. Why do most nurses wear it? The reasons may include the need for protective clothing and the need to be easily identifiable. But beyond the practicalities, nurses still cling to the traditional trappings of starched caps, cuffs and aprons at a time when many other occupational groups are abandoning or modernising their uniforms. Perhaps this love of uniform has more to do with status and group identity than it does with practical considerations or patients' needs.

Obviously, comfortable and protective clothing should be a priority for nurses. In nursing physical conditions, they need protection from bodily secretions and excretions and from contamination by bacteria. For physically strenuous work, they need comfortable clothes which enable them to lift people or bend over without hindrance or embarrassment. The patient, too, needs protection from cross-infection or from injury by unsuitable clothing or jewellery.

On both counts, however, the traditional nurse's uniform is little use, with its knee-length skirts, hats anchored on with grips, detachable cuffs and the rest. Some of the trimmings were abolished in the national uniform introduced in the 1970s, but the older-established training schools stick to their own styles of uniform as proof of higher status; as a rule, the older the school, the more fussy and impractical its uniform is.

For safety and comfort the trouser suit, worn by physiotherapists and many American nurses, is the obvious choice. Recent work on back pain, which causes at least 40 000 nurses to take a day or more off every year, shows that some of the back problems caused by lifting patients could be alleviated by wearing trousers. Abolishing the cap, which no longer prevents cross-infection or keeps hair tidy, would be another cost-saving and safety measure which would allow the nurse to think about how she is performing the lift rather than worrying about her cap falling off.

Valuable free time could also be saved by getting rid of the unnecessary paraphernalia. Changing into a fresh dress at a

London teaching hospital can take up nearly half an hour of free time — because of detachable buttons, a detachable collar, detachable apron fastenings, name badges and regalia to be transferred, and a starched muslin cap to be created anew from a flat semicircle of material. Sometimes more time is spent in school fashioning our 'dream topping' than talking about the real problems of the work.

Nevertheless many nurses are staunch defenders of their uniform, and it seems that the more traditional it is, the better they like it. In 1980 *Nursing Times* ran a competition for readers to design a 'uniform fit for the 80s', but the favourite outfits were not space-age jumpsuits or trousers, but fairly traditional dresses and caps. The winner commented that her design 'reintroduced into the uniform the femininity which most nurses feel has been lost.' It had a starched linen cap, cuffs for trained staff 'to depict status', and different coloured belts for the various grades. Other readers liked it because 'it takes the best of the traditional uniform', 'it is very feminine', and 'it makes a nurse look like a nurse, not a shop assistant or cleaner'.

Recently health authorities proposing to save money by abolishing caps have faced protests from nurses who like them — because the caps make them feel like 'real nurses'. Of course the uniform represents far more than just clothes to work in. Donning the uniform makes you part of the group, instantly recognisable as a nurse, and provides comforting security when faced with so many unknown terrors. Working your first day on a new ward or talking to an abusive drunk in the casualty department, the uniform seems to convey authority and status.

The nurse's status, as expressed in uniform, is thus made explicit to patients and to other workers (without your cap, you might be mistaken for a domestic worker). It also signifies to other nurses what position you occupy in the hierarchy. Nursing is notoriously status-conscious and goes to great lengths to show rank in the code of coloured belts, stripes on hats, badges, different coloured dresses, differently styled caps and so on. Often this makes little difference to patients, who do not always understand the symbols and who regard the nursing auxiliary as a nurse just like all the others in white caps. But nurses find great satisfaction in this authority apparel.

Progress in a nursing career tends to be described through uniform and titles rather than in relation to acquiring new skills. The extra stripe or different belt are the outward marks of increasing status, and they are seen as an end in themselves. This surely reveals a desperate insecurity. Instead of knowing who we are and what our capabilities are as individuals, we search for an identity by investing ourselves with the aura of 'nurse' through the symbolic trappings of uniform. Nurse managers of the old school continue to wear their blue dresses and lacy caps despite their lack of contact with ward work, while the more up-to-date acquire the modern management status symbols of dark suits and dictaphones.

The origins of our uniforms are also revealing. The cap may be a vestige of the veil (those of army nurses, for instance, look just like nuns) which symbolised modesty and obedience. In other ways, the uniform resembles that of other women workers in low-status service jobs, such as chambermaids and waitresses. The strings and lace tails are direct descendants of genteel Victorian headgear.

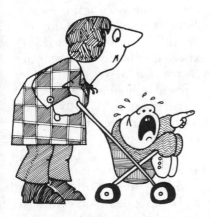 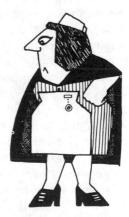

"PEOPLE REMEMBER NURSES ···"

Some people argue that uniform is reassuring for patients, a justification often used in psychiatric and mental handicap hospitals, where the traditional garb looks even more out of place. Yet the nurses who have the most confidence and independence tend to discard it or underplay it, while those who need the security of a strict hierarchy cling to it. Community nurses wear much simpler clothes. Others, like psychiatric nurses and health visitors, are abandoning uniforms because they feel it is an unnecessary barrier which emphasises separation and hinders the growth of a trusting relationship between equals. Why on earth should nurses dealing with the problems of mental illness wear aprons and hats? 'Because you couldn't tell the nurses from the patients' is the frequent answer — but would that be so terrible? If the nurse is a competent practitioner perhaps she should not need such camouflage.

Rewriting nursing history

The dichotomy between the image of nursing and the reality is currently being highlighted in another unexpected and scholarly quarter — in the field of nursing history. As we have already seen, the ruling elite of the nursing profession has, for its own ends, written or made use of a biased and inaccurate version of the history of the occupation, while today, despite the growing volume of research into the true origins of nursing, students are still given an idealised picture of past pioneers and are expected to behave in a manner which would supposedly have pleased Miss Nightingale. From Ladybird books to lectures in school, the history of nursing is presented as a pageant of great and saintly ladies, and as progress from gloomy Dickensian beginnings to our current state of supposed enlightenment.

The 'Pilgrim's Progress' view of history has been challenged in other fields by historians whose interest lies primarily in ordinary people and their lives, rather than in kings and queens and battles. It has taken some time to percolate through to nursing history, but in 1980 the publication of a collection of essays entitled *Rewriting Nursing*

History marked a breakthrough; the experience of the many is looked at, and events are placed firmly in their social and cultural context. Mick Carpenter's history of COHSE, for example, pursues a neglected thread by looking at nursing in asylums, the precursors of psychiatric hospitals — questioning the assumption that *the* history of nursing is the history of general nursing only.

Carpenter's research is also unearthing other information which sheds new light on the assumptions nurses have been encouraged to adopt about their own past. His pamphlet *All for One*, published by COHSE, describes early strikes by asylum nurses for better pay and conditions — belying the myths that industrial action is alien to nurses, or else that it is a recent phenomenon and symptom of an increasingly uncaring society. Another historian, Christopher Maggs, has looked at the previous work experience and social background of early recruits to general nursing, making us think afresh about the clichéd view of Nightingale's nurses as dedicated and well-bred young ladies.

The myths may partly have arisen because of the lack of research into nursing history. But there is also evidence to suggest that the image of nursing put forward in conventional history is not based purely on misinterpretation or ignorance; it has served a more political purpose by being used as a form of social control, reinforcing certain strands and beliefs in a tradition which has done little to protect or enhance the interests of the rank and file nurse. The gap between the image and the reality has ideological connotations in nursing history, as everywhere else.

It is not purely a fashion in history-writing which causes every nurse to know the name of Nightingale but to be ignorant of the 1922 asylum workers' strike. The authorised version of history that nurses have been given emphasises assumptions and activities which reinforce the status quo, and deliberately avoids or conceals historical evidence of discontent and pressure for change in power relations or working conditions. Perhaps it is feared that certain historical examples might put dangerous ideas into people's heads.

The reality — who we are

Trying to make sense of the data about nurses is like searching for the needle in the proverbial haystack. There are large volumes of Department of Health and Social Security statistics, but in many fields the DHSS says it cannot provide detailed information because the cost of collecting it is too great. This lack of coherent information, which may partly reflect nursing's low status, makes analysis of the occupation more difficult — it is harder to ascertain exactly who nurses are and what the reality is. The first-ever full study of the numbers of community nursing staff was only recently completed, and in some areas, such as psychiatry, there is virtually no data on who the nurses are, where they come from, their previous work experience and so on.

The figures on manpower often vary widely. Some sources distinguish between full-time and part-time workers, though usually the numbers are expressed as 'whole-time equivalents', i.e. two nurses working 37½ hours a week between them are counted as one WTE. 'Nursing staff' is usually taken to mean all Whitley Council nursing grades, which includes nursing auxiliaries and assistants, students and qualified nurses and midwives. The government, trade unions, the media and nurses themselves often fail to distinguish between qualified and unqualified staff when they talk about 'nurses' — sometimes for reasons of ideology, but sometimes through ignorance.

In the past, records held by the statutory bodies of people with qualifications such as state registration or the midwifery certificate have also been unreliable. The register of nurses held by the General Nursing Council for England and Wales, for example, included many people who were dead. However, this is being rectified with the replacement of the old statutory bodies by the UK Central Council and national boards, which are collating the records on a computer to produce an accessible and reliable list — which contains fertile information for studying nurses and their career movements.

Evidence on other subjects, such as nurses' racial origins,

is virtually non-existent. It is probably true to say, for example, that black nurses are clustered at the bottom of the hierarchy, but there is little statistical proof. Other information, such as the number of married women in nursing, is also lacking. Many staff work part-time and less is known about them. So whether we are looking at age, race, class, education, marital status, gender or sexual orientation, the reality of nurses is elusive and ill-documented.

Gender

Some information is available on the numbers of men and women in nursing, but like many of the other figures, it is patchy. The General Nursing Council documented the gender of nurses between 1955 and 1971, and although the statutory bodies no longer do this, it is possible to draw some inferences from the GNC statistics. During those years, men made up between 4·3% and 6·4% of the successful candidates for the general part of the register. Overall, though, they now comprise around 10% of the nursing workforce, a proportion which appears to be dropping despite the growing numbers of men coming into the occupation.

The percentage of men in fact varies with grade, geographical region, and specialty. Generally speaking, the more senior the grade, the greater the proportion of men: they are much more likely to stay in the profession after qualifying, and they are promoted out of all proportion to their numbers. Thus, there is only about one male to every 19 female nursing auxiliaries and assistants (1980 figures, England only); one male to every 10 female students; and one male to every five female registered nurses in all specialties. In senior jobs the figures are the most startling, with nearly half the top management and education posts occupied by men (though with enormous regional variations).

Traditionally men have tended to work in psychiatry and mental handicap, and are still clustered in those fields, although there is a drift away into general nursing. In 1971 a quarter of all registered nurses were men, but the percentage varied from 60% in mental handicap to 59% in psychiatry to only 11% in all the other fields. Interestingly, in 1970–1 over a third of the male nursing students came from overseas. At that time men occupied a third of the senior management posts, which has now risen to nearly half.

Further evidence of this male takeover (or, as has been suggested, this 'female give-away') comes in the staffing of the statutory bodies, professional organisations and trade unions, and the membership of their councils and committees. The higher echelons of the trade unions have always been dominated by men, even in the public sector unions where women make up the bulk of the membership. The Confederation of Health Service Employees, traditionally it is true a stronghold of mental nurses, has at the time of writing a male president, vice president, general secretary and deputy general secretary; only one woman holding one of six national full-time posts; no female regional secretaries; and only three women on its 28–strong executive council — yet around 78% of its members are women. The National Union of Public Employees does slightly better with 10 women on its 28–strong national executive (including five in women-only seats) and a female president, while its general secretary and 121 out of 127 regional officers are men. Women comprise 66% of the membership, and 42% of NUPE stewards.

The Royal College of Nursing did not even admit men until 1960, but they are increasingly coming to dominate the organisation, which now has its first ever male general secretary. Around half of its full-time regional and professional officers are men, as are 12 of its elected and honorary council of 28. The statutory bodies tend to show a similar picture of male over-representation. The UKCC, for example, has 26 female and 19 male members; most of the latter were appointed by the secretary of state, whereas most of the women were elected by nurses themselves. Women still hold sway in the Health Visitors Association and the Royal College of Midwives, however, since there are virtually no male practitioners in those fields yet.

Race

The lack of detailed statistical information on nurses is even more marked when it comes to race. Even before gathering information on ethnic origin came to be regarded as politically sensitive, there was almost no data, except records of the number of nursing students from overseas — which of course did not include British-born ethnic minority groups. The great local variation in numbers of British-born and migrant blacks (meaning all non-whites) makes generalisation difficult too, but there is no disputing the conclusion of a recent North London Polytechnic study — 'historically migrant workers have played an essential part in maintaining the NHS.'

Nursing was indeed one of the first occupations to look to overseas workers to boost labour shortages; the recruitment of 'aliens' as nurses began as early as 1941, and by 1948 — the year the NHS was founded — local selection committees to recruit nurses and midwives had been set up in 16 British colonies. Unemployment and the deepening crisis of racism in the 1980s are creating new and adverse conditions for migrant workers as well as for indigenous blacks, but they are still a vital part of the nursing workforce in many areas, especially in lower grades in the hierarchy and in unpopular specialties such as geriatrics and mental handicap.

The paucity of official statistics means that much information about race and employment in the NHS comes from anecdotal sources, all too easily dismissed by people who are reluctant to acknowledge the health service's pervasive, institutionalised racism. Cherrill Hicks, a journalist who carried out one of the very few investigations of racism and nursing, pinpoints the existence of two different worlds — a yawning gap between nurse managers' perception of race relations in the NHS, and the experience of black nurses themselves.

The authors of the North London Polytechnic survey assessed the official information and found very little on nurses, while neither the Salmon report nor the Briggs report, two major studies of nursing in the NHS, deals with

'When I was in the ward, doctors and visitors would walk past me looking for a white face. They'd approach a porter, an ancillary, even a patient. "Who's in charge?" they'd ask. "Where's sister?"'

Midwife

'"You people are best fitted to do practical nursing," I've heard the director of nurse education say. Or, "When these people are given a chance they do work hard." He doesn't even remember I'm one of them.'

Tutor

'If we get one or two of us at sister level we're meant to be grateful. I personally think they have a quota on how many blacks they employ in particular posts.'

Health visitor

From Hicks C. (1982). Racism in Nursing. *Nursing Times*; **78 (18):** 743–48.

overseas nurses in any detail. Organisations like the UK Council for Overseas Student Affairs have data collected for specific practical purposes, but 'we still have no idea about the total number of overseas-born nurses in the NHS', and of course still less about indigenous non-white nurses.

The data unearthed on nurses in training showed that in 1977 nearly 12% of students and pupils had been born overseas (66% from the Commonwealth, 22% from Ireland and 11% from elsewhere). Within the Commonwealth, the largest category was Malaysians (a fifth of the total), followed by West Indians (15%) and Mauritians (8%), with Filipinos accounting for 4%. The numbers coming from abroad to train reached a peak in 1970 and are falling sharply. As a percentage of all nursing students, those born overseas vary between only 2·3% in the Northern RHA to 34% in the North East Thames RHA; they are also distributed unevenly within authorities, being more likely to work in mental and geriatric hospitals.

This pattern may well be repeated among qualified staff but there is no evidence, even of the numbers involved. These may be affected by the fact that nurses who entered the UK on student visas to do their training are now being refused work permits if they decide they want to stay; unemployment is hitting this group even harder than the rest, for health authorities who do not have the money to offer posts to newly qualified nurses are tending to avoid the bureaucratic problems of work permits — and the overseas nurse's loss of the job means losing the right to stay in the UK.

Another trend is the likelihood that black recruits, wherever they were born, are encouraged to undertake training for enrolment rather than registration — even though they may have the necessary qualifications to enter the registration programme. Those recruited abroad may not be aware of the difference, but it not only deprives them ultimately of the chance of promotion in UK hospitals, but may bar them from nursing work in their own countries, as in the Philippines where the EN is not a recognised qualification. Hard evidence is lacking but black nurses claim that channelling them into EN training is a covert form of racism.

Other anecdotal evidence suggests that black nurses face repeated job rejection, difficulties in getting accepted for post-basic courses, and little hope of promotion. The North London Polytechnic survey of one large hospital found, for example, that West Indians were over-represented in lower grades — 61% of auxiliaries, 38% of enrolled nurses and pupils, but only 12% of registered nurses and students. Comparatively few were appointed to senior grades, although they stayed in their jobs longer and were on average older than other staff.

Many factors apart from direct discrimination might also be relevant, such as education, ability to speak the language of the dominant culture, the local labour market and so on. But the evidence all points to the existence of widespread institutional racism in the NHS; and as the 1981 riots demonstrated, any comfortable belief that the UK is happily and multiracially harmonious is misplaced. Despite strong statements from black nurses themselves and the signs of deepening discrimination, the NHS and nursing in particular have made almost no effort to promote anti-racist policies and practices.

Some schools of nursing are incorporating into the curriculum sessions on 'ethnic minorities' and the 'problems' they present as patients — well-meaning efforts, perhaps, but which all too often reinforce the idea of white English middle-class values and customs as the norm. The critical and scornful attitude of some senior nurses to ethnic dress and hairstyle shows the absence of real and positive acceptance of racial difference, even in a supposedly humane profession. In one notorious case, a school of nursing tried to bar a Sikh girl from training because she wore trousers to cover her legs in line with religious custom — telling her that 'breaking the rules' like this might lead to anarchy. A student nurse from the Caribbean was threatened with dismissal unless she stopped wearing her hair in plaits, again using the norm of 'good behaviour' as an insidious form of racial control. Again, academic work on overseas nurses has drawn attention to their 'communication problems' — though in some hospitals the white, traditional English-speaking patient might be in the minority, and the 'overseas' nurses more in tune with the needs of the majority.

The racism inherent in the NHS can be partly tackled by race awareness courses, such as those run by the group Training in Health and Race and promoted by enlightened schools and trade unions like NUPE, by comprehensive and committed health authority policies and by stronger legal back-up. Equally important, nurses can begin to recognise and combat the racism within themselves, which taints their relationships with black colleagues and patients and causes such distress. The Black Health Workers and Patients Group, founded to support black workers in their struggles and to monitor racist health policies, quotes the experience of a black nurse listening to racist 'jokes' made by a senior nurse during the ward report. 'I get used to these remarks,' she said. 'I guess hearing such remarks about "us" makes me realise my position in this society. It is my duty as a black nurse to help my black people, because the white nursing profession don't give a damn for us.'

Part-time and agency nurses

The popular image of the nurse, whether she is an angel, battleaxe or tart, is still that of an unmarried woman. Yet, as Alison Tierney recently pointed out in one of the few studies of married women in nursing, it is 'a predominantly female profession dependent for its labour force largely upon married women' — and largely on part-time workers, at that.

The picture of nursing of course reflects the national tendency for the majority of part-time workers to be women. A surprisingly large 37% of the whole nursing workforce in England in 1980 were part-timers. (See Fig. 2.1.) Tierney also draws attention to the fact that part-time nurses are concentrated almost exclusively in the lowest grades, sometimes even outnumbering the full-timers. In Scotland in the early 1970s, three-quarters of nurse administrators were single;

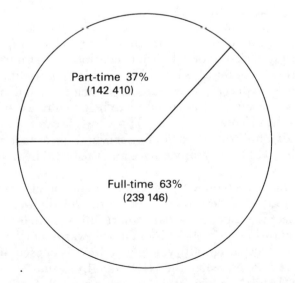

Part-time 37%
(142 410)

Full-time 63%
(239 146)

Fig. 2.1   *Full-time and part-time nursing staff in the NHS, England, 1980.*

half the sisters, and only a fifth of the staff nurses. Clearly there is some element of the chicken and the egg; women who marry and have children have less time to devote to their careers, and receive little support when it comes to flexible working hours, facilities for child care, or sharing out domestic labour.

Part-time nurses, like other part-time women workers, endure the usual disadvantages of low pay, job insecurity, lack of fringe benefits and poor promotion prospects. They are also discriminated against in professional development and continuing education. Nursing journals, books, reports, and professional and statutory bodies all propound the ideology of nursing as a profession with skilled practitioners needing constantly to update their knowledge, yet the plight of the part-timer is rarely considered despite her major role in providing nursing care. She is nearly always at the end of the queue for courses or study leave, for example. As Tierney says, 'the need is not just to employ nurses on a part-time basis, but somehow to integrate them more fully into the total workforce, by providing incentives and training opportunities which will both raise job satisfaction and the value of their contribution.'

The large numbers of part-time nurses also have implications for the new ideas about nursing care which emphasise a close, intimate relationship between individual nurses and patients. Of course this is not impossible for part-timers, but it may easily fragment the care, involving more staff, and the tendency is often for part-timers to be given more mundane and task-orientated work. Those who desire to move towards a fully qualified nursing service appear to ignore the working realities of many nurses and the NHS, in this field as in others.

Agency nurses often suffer a similar fate, being given more bitty and less interesting work — or, on the other hand, being sent to 'special' a particularly ill or difficult patient, often knowing little about them or the ward. They are often spoken of disparagingly, yet agency work is chosen by many because it offers what the NHS usually cannot — flexible hours. It enables women with children or dependent relatives to choose their working hours to fit in with other commitments.

The other major reason why people do agency work, according to a recent survey by the British Nursing Association — a large agency — is money. Nearly a quarter of nurses in the survey already had NHS jobs, and moonlighting is a common means of supplementing meagre pay to buy 'extras' such as clothes or holidays. What agency staff do not get, of course, is job security, sick pay, paid compassionate leave, maternity leave or other NHS benefits such as free uniforms or subsidised accommodation.

Some health authorities run their own 'nurse banks' which provide a pool of nurses known to the hospital or unit who can be called on to fill gaps caused by holidays or sickness. The idea was promoted by Labour health minister Barbara Castle in the 1970s, but never took off in a big way. For both hospital and nurse, however, it offers the benefits of familiarity with the environment, staff and patients, and avoids the all too common experience of being flung in at the deep end in situations the agency nurse feels ill equipped to handle. DHSS guidelines say agency nurses should be given full introductions and briefings from senior nurses, but often this doesn't happen.

Agency nursing is a frequent source of political dispute because it is seen as a substitute for good staffing levels; instead of employing enough nurses to cope with absence, authorities prefer the stopgap measure of taking on agency staff, a cheaper option but hardly one which promotes high standards of care or safeguards the welfare of individual nurses. But whatever the political arguments, there are clearly very many nurses, often married with children, who are forced into this kind of work because their needs are ignored by the NHS and by nursing's leaders — the majority of whom are men or single women.

Different types of nursing

As we saw, the typical nurse is supposed to work in an acute hospital, where patients come in with specific illnesses of the body and go home cured. Even people with inside knowledge often fall into the trap of equating 'the profession' with general hospital nurses; nursing students on general training courses may be unaware that there are separate programmes for nursing the mentally ill, the mentally handicapped, and children; in the public mind, the NHS tends to mean operations and ambulances.

Once again, looking at the statistics reminds us of realities which tend to be ignored. The information summarised in the pie charts not only tells us about the numbers of people doing different kinds of nursing, but also highlights how NHS facilities are distributed between the various categories of people who use the service. A quarter of all hospital beds are allocated to people with mental illnesses, with mentally handicapped people occupying 14% of the beds. Geriatric and young disabled people account for another 16%, and maternity for 5% — leaving less than half the beds for acute medicine and surgery (see Fig. 2.2). Bed numbers are a very crude measure of how services are used, but they do give a

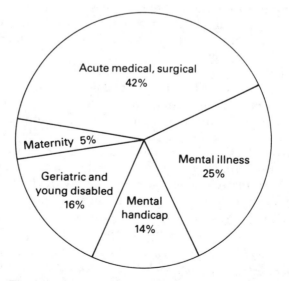

Fig. 2.2   *The average daily allocation of hospital in-patient beds in the NHS, England, 1980. Note: The percentages given in Figs. 2.2–2.5 are approximated to the nearest whole number.*

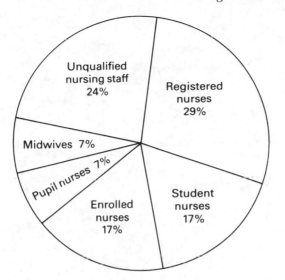

Fig. 2.3　*The distribution of nursing staff in the NHS in England in 1980, in hospitals other than mental illness and mental handicap (whole time equivalents).*

rough guide, and help to shatter the myths about what the NHS actually does. The popular emphasis on acute medicine and surgery masks the enormous need for care in the less glamorous, often long-stay areas, and use of community services is even harder to highlight since there are no bed numbers — yet for the vast majority of people it is their first, often only point of contact with health workers.

Comparing the numbers of nurses in each field with the numbers of beds (taken as a crude indication of need), big disparities appear (see Figs. 2.3, 2.4 and 2.5). There are many reasons why people's health needs and the allocation of resources do not match, but what concerns us here is the way in which those nurses who work in the less popular and most under-resourced sectors tend to suffer from similar neglect, even from other nurses. In recent years community nurses have complained bitterly about this. While they have some justification, they at least tend to have a background in general training. The isolation of psychiatric and mental handicap nurses is even greater and can partly be traced

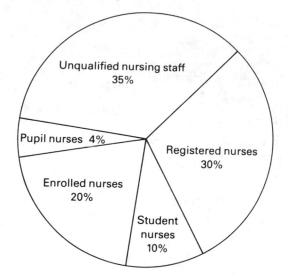

Fig. 2.4   *The distribution of nursing staff in the NHS in England in 1980, in mental illness and mental handicap hospitals (whole time equivalents).*

back to the roots of their occupations, which evolved from the asylum and poor law workers and entailed not only a different type of work from that carried out by nurses in general hospitals, but also attracted a different type of recruit.

These old schisms are no longer so acute, but there is still a marked sense of disparity, a strong feeling of separateness and difference. General nursing has always been the dominant culture in the profession, as it is now, and the lack of attention paid to mental nursing reflects the power structures in nursing as well as the social tendency to ignore the uncomfortable existence of people with 'abnormal' mental conditions. Moreover, mental nurses have usually worked in isolated institutions — the large, long-stay asylums locked away from the world, largely self-sufficient and employing whole village populations — which have kept them apart from the opportunity to share their concerns with others in the mainstream of professional and health care politics.

This isolation is gradually breaking down, as new policies

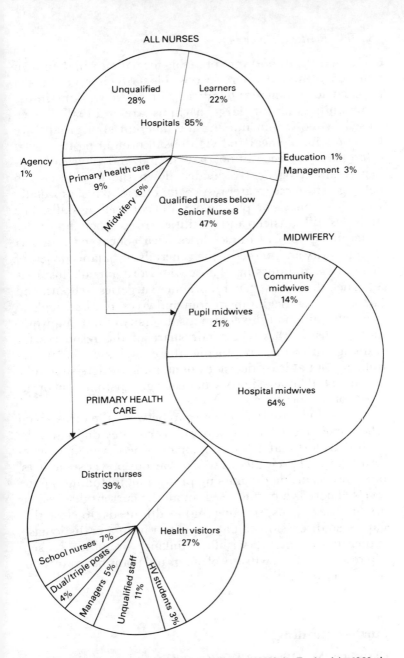

Fig. 2.5 *The distribution of nursing staff in the NHS in England in 1980, by grades and within specialties (whole time equivalents).*

emphasise the importance of caring for patients in their own home environment wherever possible. Growing numbers of psychiatric and mental handicap nurses are working in the community and the large asylums are gradually being closed, while within nursing the different staff groups are becoming more vocal and vigorous in promoting their own interests. The recognition that mental and physical well-being cannot be neatly divided down the middle is also helping to foster a greater respect for others' skills, especially with the emphasis on psychology and counselling skills. The divisions still run deep and hostilities are common, however.

Several groups of nurses have been concerned to assert their identity and to rectify the generally unbalanced view of health care and nursing. Those who work outside hospitals — in health centres, general practice surgeries, schools, and factories — are beginning to join midwives in the struggle to gain recognition of the enormous diversity of nursing work, and to ensure they get a fair share of the resources for training and care. Balancing these demands is always difficult, but at least decisions by nursing leaders should be based on full knowledge of what each group does, and of the needs of its clients.

To conclude, there is a huge gap between the ideas about who nurses are, what they do and where they do it, and the reality. Unfortunately that gap, maintained by media misinformation and prejudice as well as various power structures, often yawns inside the nursing profession, including the top levels. There is a crying need, in all the current discussions about future plans, training and health needs, to close that gap — so discussion can at least start from a realistic base, rather than fantasy, wishful thinking, prejudice or self-interest. Only then will any of our grand plans have any hope of coming to fruition.

Further Reading

Carpenter M. (1980). *All for One*. Banstead: Confederation of Health Service Employees.

Davies C. ed. (1980). *Rewriting Nursing History*. London: Croom Helm.

Doyal L. *et al.* (1980). *Migrant Workers in the NHS — report of a preliminary survey*. London: Department of Sociology, Polytechnic of North London.

Hicks C. (1982). Racism in Nursing. *Nursing Times*; May 5, pp. 743–8 and May 12, pp. 789–91.

Hughes J., McNaught A., Pennell I. (eds) (1984). *Race and Employment in the NHS*. London: King Edward's Hospital Fund for London.

Kalisch B., Kalisch P., Scobey M. (1983). *Images of the Nurse on Television*. New York: Springer.

Maggs C. (1983). *The Origins of General Nursing*. London: Croom Helm.

Mills & Boon (publishers). Any novel in the 'Doctor-Nurse Romance' series, eg. *Wish with the Candles* by Betty Neels, *The Doctor's Decision* by Elizabeth Petty.

Muff J. ed. (1982). *Socialization, Sexism and Stereotyping — women's issues in nursing*. St. Louis: C. V. Mosby.

Nuttall P. (1983). Male Takeover or Female Giveaway? *Nursing Times*; January 12, pp. 10–11.

Salvage J. (1982). Angles not Angels. *The Health Services*, September 3.

Tierney A. (1983). Married Women in Nursing. *Nursing Times*, Occasional Paper, September 7.

The source for the information in Figs. 2.1–2.5 is: DHSS (1982). *Health and Personal Social Services Statistics for England 1982*. London: HMSO.

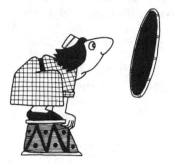

3

Through the hoops

The two or three years spent training for a statutory nursing qualification have an enormous influence on the kind of work nurses do, and the way they do it. From the moment the new recruit sets foot in the school of nursing, she is encouraged to put on not only a uniform but a whole set of attitudes to her role and her work, and she is subjected to a whole new range of powerful, formative influences. Many of these are not as obvious or explicit as the content of classroom sessions or clinical experiences, but this 'hidden curriculum' is equally important and influential.

The 'making of a nurse' has many facets. What she is taught — or not taught — in the classroom, the observations she makes of how care is actually given in the wards or community, and the values and assumptions of her teachers and the institution all help to determine what kind of nurse she will be. When thinking about the reforms needed in nursing education — and everyone agrees they are badly needed — it is important to look not just at courses and curricula but at all these different influences. Trying to make big changes by tackling only one isolated aspect will have only limited results. Professionalism, the nursing hierarchy, and learning and teaching methods are just as crucial as the model syllabuses drawn up by the statutory training bodies.

Nurses — made or born?

Is it possible to make someone into a good nurse through training and if so, how? This argument has raged ever since nursing was first established as an occupation. Some people believe 'good nurses' have the right qualities through instinct, luck or an accident of birth, and need only a bare minimum of instruction, while others think nursing should be a graduate profession with every nurse taking a degree. Yet others believe the decision to be a nurse implies an attempt to fulfil deep psychological/emotional needs.

But despite these contrasting views, and the enormous changes in our health care system during the course of this century, nursing training seems to have altered remarkably little. The current three-year route to registration, with its emphasis on learning in the clinical setting backed up by relatively short periods of formal teaching, is not very different from that of 1925, when the General Nursing Council of England and Wales held its first state final examinations. Students were really workers whose educational needs were secondary to their value as cheap labour. Teaching methods were unimaginative, relying on rote learning rather than individual development. Medical knowledge, rather than nursing, dominated the syllabus.

Unfortunately there is much evidence that those criticisms are still true today. Changing such an entrenched system is hard, especially when there is a serious shortage of teachers and ward staff in many areas, leaving the student to fend for herself — but there are hopeful signs of improvement, not least the now common recognition that much is wrong with nursing education. Some senior nurses are working against the odds to support their students with stimulating and thoughtful teaching, trying out new approaches and thinking up new ideas. Yet it still appears to be an uphill struggle.

Student status

Nursing students today (i.e. students and pupils — those in training for registration or enrolment by a statutory body) make up at least a quarter of the nursing workforce in the NHS. Very often they are students in name only, for in hospitals with training schools attached they often comprise the bulk of the labour force. They may be called on to take charge of the ward, move without notice to an unfamiliar ward, work split shifts or change their days off — all to fit in with the hospital's needs, not their own. And having finished a tiring day's work, they are expected to study for exams and complete assignments set by the school in their time off.

The nursing student has a hard life compared with university or college undergraduates. Doing her studying on top of a mentally and physically draining job, with a number of weeks a year spent in school and four or five on holiday, leaves little time for the other activities which enable college students to relax and develop new interests. While other students may be acting in plays, working for the students' union or mixing with people in a variety of disciplines, nursing students are swotting for exams or recovering from night duty.

Some universities and polytechnics now offer degree courses in nursing, or a degree course in a relevant subject which may be combined with nursing training based at a nearby hospital. Students still have to fulfil the statutory nursing requirements in order to qualify, but they can at least get a taste of the advantages of college life and the broadening of scope it can bring. However, nurses graduating from such courses are a tiny minority, and public spending cuts are threatening the future of some departments.

Nursing training is ultimately the responsibility of special bodies established by law to protect the public. The primary duty of the UK Central Council for Nursing, Midwifery and Health Visiting and the national boards for England, Scotland, Wales and Northern Ireland is to ensure that the public is looked after by safe practitioners; this is enacted through rules governing nursing education and the conduct of qualified and student staff. Only by conforming to these rules is the nurse legally allowed to practise.

With their legal control of the admission of students to the professional register (defining them as qualified nurses),

'I was lucky with my first ward allocation. It was a medical ward where many of the patients were old hands and had been admitted before — especially in the winter when their bronchitis was bad and their homes were cold and damp — so they knew the ropes and were a great help to frightened new students like me.

We were also lucky to have a friendly, energetic and caring charge nurse. Everyone was on first name terms, the atmosphere was happy despite the enormous workload, and he was respected by everyone for his willingness to pitch in and do the work — unlike other ward sisters who seemed to prefer chatting to the doctors over endless cups of tea in their out-of-bounds offices. There was an open and inquiring approach to nursing care and students, auxiliaries and patients were all encouraged to ask questions and discuss problems.

This questioning attitude was something I took for granted from my university background — it's the best way to learn — and I enjoyed my time on the ward, despite the traumas of seeing people suffering and dying. So I was a bit taken aback when it came to receiving my ward report. "I've enjoyed having you here and I appreciate your enthusiasm and your desire to learn about nursing through questions and discussions," the charge nurse told me. "But a word of warning — I like this, but many others don't. So be careful not to ask too many questions, because there are a lot of people who will resent you for it."

I couldn't believe my ears, but how right he was. My awakening was rude in all senses of the word. On my next allocation the ward sister's approach to students was to bellow abuse at them across the ward for their "misdemeanours", in the hearing of all the patients, and to send them crying into the sluice after a verbal lashing.'

SRN, London

these bodies lay down the framework and content of training. They can stipulate, for example, how much time must be spent in each specialty (incorporating rules laid down by the European Community), how much night duty should be worked and what subjects should be covered in the curricula. They also inspect schools of nursing and the related clinical workplaces to ensure that they provide an adequate and appropriate learning environment, and the statutory bodies can close a training school if it is below standard. Potentially this is a powerful measure, and can be used as a way of enforcing improvements, for many hospitals rely on students to maintain their workforce; if student intakes were stopped, wards might have to be closed, putting the hospital in a difficult and embarrassing position.

Although the nursing profession therefore possesses some means of controlling training and establishing its own standards, there is little uniformity. Standards vary enormously from one school to the next and in some places are abysmal. Recruitment policies, health authority resources and attitudes all make an immense difference. Some schools, such as those attached to major teaching hospitals, are flooded with applications and can therefore demand high entrance requirements, while others — especially those offering mental handicap and mental illness training in large, isolated hospitals — keep requirements to the statutory minimum in the struggle to attract staff. And like entrance requirements, the quality of teaching and ward experience is variable, between and within institutions.

In theory the statutory bodies could use their powers much more forcefully to raise standards. Yet in practice even

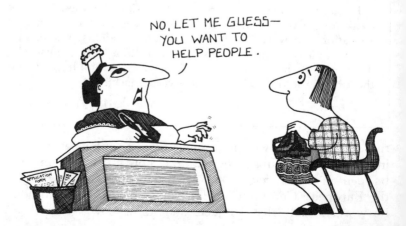

their duty to protect the public is often neglected, with seriously ill people left in the care of students who are too ill-prepared or inexperienced to nurse safely. It is surprising that more mistakes don't happen; and such situations threaten the morale and confidence of the student as well as the welfare of the patient. The problem is that nominal powers are useless unless there is the money, the authority and the will to use them. Despite its importance, nursing has always been subordinate in the NHS and has failed to claim or win the resources it needs. But it must also be said that the statutory bodies, although they may lack such powers, have failed to exploit their legal responsibilities to the full and to fight tooth and nail for the profession. A new order may be beginning with the newly established UKCC and boards, but it remains to be seen whether they will fight for nursing more courageously and independently than their forebears.

The nursing student, then, is not really a student but a worker. Like apprentices in other occupations, she is badly paid and has little status, yet she lacks the close supervision by experts inherent in the true apprenticeship system. She does not enjoy the same rights as qualified nurses or auxiliary workers, and employment law takes no account of her anomalous position — yet she is not protected as a student either. She is obliged to conform to the statutory rules, which may, for example, deny her the right to refuse to take part in treatment she considers to be unethical. In 1982 psychiatric students in at least three hospitals were sacked for refusing to take part in sessions of electroconvulsive therapy (ECT), because they disagreed in principle with the use of a treatment whose effects can be harmful and whose operation is not scientifically understood. By refusing to do it they failed to conform to the training rules as interpreted by their schools, and therefore lost their livelihood and future career.

No-one is happy with the current position of nursing students, and there have been various proposals to give them full student status, or else call them 'protected employees' with contracts which take account of their special position. But such ideas have been around for some time, and nothing has been done. Other urgent matters always seem to be more

'Our training actively discourages us from discussing our work critically and encourages us to view our problems as individual failings. The classic incident occurred two wards back when sister took me into her office the day before I was due to leave, to ask me how I felt about the ward. She had decided I must be very unhappy as I did not appear to smile much, when in fact I had been perfectly content, though extremely harassed most of the time "trying to get the work done". So she asked me my thoughts — and I told her. Sister listened attentively, though her face grew more and more stern, so I knew she was not taking kindly to what I said. She sharply asked how I could improve the situation, so I tentatively suggested that a bit more organisation was needed. My reply from her was to the effect that I only had ten months' nursing experience, compared with her ten years, so anything I said was worthless and not worth discussing further. The following day I collected my report and discovered that I am a quiet, dour girl with little enthusiasm or motivation who is too critical of the running of the ward. It was at this stage that I could easily have packed it in because of my feelings of frustration and helplessness.'

SRN

The ideal recruit

A famous specialist hospital in London, when requesting references for potential new nursing staff, sends out a pre-printed letter to referees stating that 'good health is essential, a good education, also intelligence and common sense.'

It goes on: 'It is desirous that members of the nursing staff should be of a patient, cheerful and kindly disposition, willing and able to apply themselves to their studies, and amenable to a reasonable degree of discipline.'

The letter then asks for assessments of the applicant under these headings: general temperament and disposition, intelligence and capabilities, moral character.

pressing — and there is one factor which probably counts for more than all the rest: the shortage of trained staff. In 1972 the Briggs committee said students 'should not consider themselves as nor be considered as part of the ordinary labour force of the NHS', and the idea that students should be supernumerary has been stressed by all the organisations, but nothing has happened. If students really were to be supplementary to staffing needs, there would have to be a huge increase in nursing labour — especially in trained staff to give supervision and teaching as well as care. Students' learning experiences would be carefully planned and supervised, and more staff would be needed to perform some of the jobs they now do.

There is no sign that any government is prepared to invest in health care the large sums such a change would entail. Nurses are slow to push their claims and there is no support from doctors. In fact, the goal of student status is now so far from realisation that the statutory bodies, retreating from the Briggs position, are talking about 'protected employee' status instead. This might clear up some problems, but it would not solve the major problem of trainees often being expected to carry the responsibilities of qualified nurses.

The bodies are proposing a new structure for nursing and its implications are only slowly becoming apparent. They intend to abolish enrolled nurse training and prepare all students for registration, giving qualified staff a supervisory role over students, with many tasks to be performed by untrained 'care assistants' (removing the 'nursing' from the auxiliary's title). There is talk of designated wards for training, special preparation for staff nurses and sisters, and more ward-based teaching — but little talk of the cost implications. It seems that the only feasible way to introduce such ideas without extra resources is to train fewer nurses — which offers a bleak future to hospitals which already have recruitment problems and whose work is mostly done by untrained staff. Greater burdens will be loaded on the auxiliary staff, an irony since they are regarded by the nursing establishment as being incapable of giving a high standard of care without very close supervision.

This policy of the statutory bodies is complementary in most respects to the model proposed by the RCN in its reports on standards of care and the nursing career structure. The changes have not been spelled out very explicitly, nor yet accepted as broad patterns for the future, yet some alterations are going ahead piecemeal, such as the phasing out of enrolled nurse training. There is great uncertainty, fuelled by an apparent reluctance or inability to describe simply and clearly what the changes will mean (the bodies themselves are in any case hampered by drastic money problems). Today's students will complete their training in the old way, but as qualified staff they may well have to incorporate some new ideas into their work.

Who helps the student?

None of the nursing organisations has much to be proud of in its support for nursing students, whose problems have largely been ignored. Students belonging to the RCN (making up a third of the membership) have their own association, but the organisation has not always thrown its full weight behind them. The generic trade unions often neglect to recruit student nurses (and are anyway often blocked in their efforts by obstructive schools of nursing who do not consider trade union membership to be appropriate), and fail to concentrate on their special needs.

Students who want to question or comment on what happens in their school or hospital have a difficult time. They are often viewed with suspicion and hostility by senior nurses, many of whom trained at a time when students, and perhaps women in general, were expected to be seen and not heard on sensitive or controversial issues. Open discussion itself tends to be seen as criticism and those who ask the questions are labelled as trouble-makers; questioning, criticism and conflict are not regarded as healthy, but as threatening.'If you wanted to think, you shouldn't have come into nursing' sums up the attitude of many senior staff, in education or service.

Those students who feel bound to raise issues which are

'Practical work conditions left me feeling pressured and stressed. Staff shortages upset me the most, since it meant I was unavoidably compromised into giving inadequate care. In the mad rush to do all the jobs it was impossible to talk to patients other than superficially, and horrible to discover later that a patient had felt he or she could not approach a nurse "because you were so busy". As a student nurse during my psychiatric secondment I asked, on ethical grounds, not to have anything to do with ECT. The director of nursing education gave me a counselling session about this, during which she said: "Who do you think you are to question the doctors? If you wanted to think, you should not have come into nursing." Ironically, it is because I wanted to remain "caring" that I left nursing. Trying to care in the present system was a little like being flung in at the deep end with weights round my neck and told to swim. I think many nurses are in fact drowning, not waving, even if they have fixed smiles on their faces.'

SRN, London

worrying them — whether it concerns the care on a particular ward, teaching problems or conditions of work — are in a vulnerable position. Successfully completing your training depends partly on having good ward reports, and it is felt (though impossible to prove) that those who ask 'too many' questions may have a bad report for their pains, thus jeopardising their future. At a time when jobs for newly qualified staff are harder to come by and nurses are facing redundancies, the pressure to keep quiet is even greater. And even if it is only a minority of senior staff who would allow their prejudices to put a student's future at risk, there is a strong feeling that anonymous conformity is safe, while assertive or questioning behaviour is dangerous.

People who want to express their views — and nearly everyone at some time feels strongly about something — might think twice about it in these circumstances. But if you are aware of the pitfalls and of your rights, it can be done — especially if the views come from a group rather than an individual. One person can be ignored but it is more difficult to write off a group of 10, 20 or 30. At one geriatric hospital, some students on secondment noticed that patients were being ill-treated; everyone had actually known for some time how bad things were, but nothing was done until a group of students decided they would all approach their school with written and oral evidence of what was happening. No single person could be made a scapegoat and the protest could not easily be ignored. With trade union advice, the students took good care to keep copies of all correspondence and statements they made; the outcome was a promise to make improvements.

Trade unions

Everyone is entitled to join a union and student nurses are no exception. Often representatives from the RCN, COHSE and NUPE are asked to talk to groups of new students and offer them membership, but some schools are in the habit of forgetting to invite the TUC unions, thus ensuring that most people join the RCN (occasionally the reverse happens in psychiatric schools and the college does not get a look in). If such a session is scheduled, students should find out which other unions have a branch at the hospital and make sure a representative attends the session — this will give people a better opportunity to compare what the organisations have to offer and to decide which one they want to join, if any.

The TUC unions all have well-developed networks of stewards who can advise nurses and inform them of their rights. Often, though not always, the steward will be a nurse and there may be a special nurses' section of the union with its own meetings. The full-time officers usually have plenty of experience in dealing with managers on a variety of matters — even those which might not be thought of as industrial relations; though some lack knowledge of nursing matters, this may be compensated by their negotiating skills and thorough knowledge of employment law and Whitley Council conditions.

Professional organisations

The RCN, with some 55 000 student members, has its own Association of Nursing Students (ANS) with an elected national committee, paid full-time officers, and representatives on the college's policy-making council. Some hospitals have RCN 'student units' which meet regularly to discuss matters of concern and interest, and nationally the ANS has tried to highlight problems such as poor accommodation and the unfair treatment of students who fail their exams.

No other organisation has a service aimed specifically at nursing students, so the RCN might appear to be the obvious one to join, but there is one big problem. This is the fact that the senior education or service nurses to or about whom the student might want to complain are often themselves RCN members — causing divided loyalties if outside advice or representation is needed. The presence of managers at RCN meetings may also blunt the edge of legitimate criticisms by junior staff, as well as diluting the actions the groups might take on issues like cuts or job losses.

Student councils

Many training schools have councils of representatives from each set, which meet to discuss relevant matters. They usually report directly to the director of nurse education (DNE) and are a good forum in which to raise problems of all kinds, although they do not have any real power. People tend not to see the councils as useful or relevant, and it is important to make sure they really do address themselves to the issues everyone grumbles about round the canteen table. In schools which do not have a council, students could start one by talking to their set and enlisting the help and advice of a sympathetic tutor. Like all such committees it can only be effective with good support and commitment, but where this is forthcoming the DNE is bound to pay some attention to it.

Support groups

These have developed more recently as an answer to the lack

of opportunity in nursing to share problems and feelings about the job. People meet informally and talk about whatever interests or bothers them, and often find comfort and support from sharing their feelings; sometimes the groups may also get involved in activities such as pay campaigns or local opposition to NHS cuts. Sometimes they exist under the wing of a union, but most are open to anyone; anyone can start one. Some of the nurses' support groups are linked nationally through the Radical Nurses Group, which holds regular conferences where people meet to talk about nursing, and can also give advice to people who want to start new groups in their own hospitals.

'I had gone into midwifery with a vague idea that it would somehow be an independent, interesting and different sort of job and I wanted to be with women. I believed I would have the power to change the bad experiences of childbirth which my friends had told me about. Well, my illusions were soon dispelled during the first weeks when I was literally thrown on to the labour wards. I was untrained and nervous. The only previous training they had given us was six weeks of general nursing in the classroom which had little to do with midwifery. Yet on the wards nobody showed me anything. Nobody had the time. There was always an acute shortage of staff. Sometimes I would work on the labour and antenatal wards where there were two wards with eight women in labour and six other patients. We literally had to run up and down those corridors. The work was killing and there were always pressures on us to work harder. Yet we were supposed to grit our teeth and carry on in these gruelling conditions without complaining, always smiling, calm, "professional" and subservient. In fact most of us hated the work and we were always talking about leaving, but we had no choice but to go on. We came from the West Indies, Malaysia, Ireland, Africa and India and we had little money. They had us trapped.'

Midwife, London

The content of nursing education

Some of the impetus behind nursing training in its early days — and much of its content — came from the upsurge of interest in medicine as a science. Although nurses controlled the patient's environment through housekeeping duties, they were also expected to act as medical assistants, and much of their formal training took the form of lectures from doctors. Even now many nursing schools invite hospital consultants to lecture on medical specialties, while until recently most conferences on nursing, and the nursing journals, involved much medical participation. Doctors have also had a powerful influence on the occupation through their membership of nursing committees, statutory bodies and even selection panels, an arrangement which for the most part is not reciprocated.

Today, however, more and more people are beginning to recognise that medicine is only one of many factors which affect health and that, in spite of its brilliant successes, medicine cannot provide all the answers to ill health. The nurse as the health worker involved in most aspects of care — including assessment, diagnosis, treatment, rehabilitation, pain relief and nutrition, let alone preventing disease — is able to survey the entire spectrum and to appreciate that the medical approach is only part of the solution to the problems of preventing and treating illness and maintaining good health. It might therefore be expected that nursing education would be based on a broad overview, incorporating knowledge from many disciplines. But on the whole training is still dominated by the medical model of illness, which sees the body primarily as a collection of organs to be serviced ('cured') when something breaks down.

Many schools, however, and indeed the new curricula produced by the statutory bodies, are now beginning to emphasise the need for nursing, as opposed to medical, knowledge. Yet this creates new problems, for while second-hand medicine may no longer be appropriate, there is no consensus yet about what nursing knowledge actually is. But whether it is a separate discipline or a combination of knowledge from many fields, there is a growing agreement that the medical model is only of limited use in patient care. A working knowledge of basic anatomy and physiology is still thought to be essential; psychology and an understanding of the social, economic and environmental factors which affect the health of individuals and society are coming to be seen as equally vital aspects of the nurse's knowledge. Good nursing is not inferior or second-hand medicine, but demands different skills. Nurses need to know the physiological causes of, say, bedsores, not only to heal them but to ensure that nursing care is based on an intelligent strategy to prevent them. If there is only limited time to learn all this, it is more important to know how effectively to intervene than to be able to recite the Latinate names of the layers of the skin. Knowing the body mechanisms does not solve the bedsores problem, and since the doctor has that knowledge, the nurse should perhaps concentrate on other things in her sphere: is the sore partly the result of dietary deficiencies in the hospital food? Are there enough staff to ensure the patient is turned often? If nurses don't ask such questions, no-one else will, and knowing what and whom to ask is more important to the nurse's work than knowing the intricacies of the islets of Langerhans or the signs and symptoms of pernicious anaemia.

Some schools are thinking along the lines of nursing as a discrete discipline and base their teaching on the various 'models of nursing' developed in recent years. These look at nursing as a set of specific activities in its own right, not as a medical assistant job simply carrying out orders, and suggest different approaches to patient care which emphasise the individuality of each person and the need to tailor their care to their personal requirements — taking into account not just pathology but personality, environment, social class and much else. The models are sometimes dismissed as 'just theory', but they are actually much more firmly rooted in practice than the gallop through the body's physiological systems which is still the basis of so much nursing education.

All students today will come across the nursing process, which exemplifies the belief in nursing as a discipline in its own right. Much mumbo-jumbo has crept into discussion of the process since its arrival from the USA, but its basis is simple — a planned and systematic approach to care involving assessing the patient's needs, planning the care, giving it and then evaluating how successful it was. The heated arguments and reams of care plans, histories and charts have obscured the fact that it is a tool and not the answer to every problem.

The confusion and hostility surrounding the nursing process demonstrates how care cannot be separated from other influences, and how nursing education is tied up with the rest of the occupation. On the one hand, people who believe nursing has a claim to be a profession have seized on the process as a way of establishing autonomy, as it appears to offer a scientific approach to nursing care which counterbalances medical prescription. It is also a useful way of differentiating qualified from auxiliary staff, as only trained staff are held to be responsible for supervising the process, and it is thus a useful tactic in the professionalism war. On the other hand, it has met with much opposition because of the insensitive and autocratic way in which some senior nurses have tried to introduce it, imposing it on the staff often with scant understanding of what it is about, which inevitably produces resentment. Change forced from above is usually unwelcome.

The syllabus

Ground rules for the syllabuses are laid down by the statutory bodies in accordance with European Community directives (ensuring that nursing qualifications in EC member countries will be interchangeable). The required experience for general nursing training is now extensive, including general and specialist medicine, general and specialist surgery, child care and paediatrics, maternity care, mental health and psychiatry, care of the elderly and geriatrics, and home nursing/community work. The new mental illness and mental handicap syllabuses, introduced in 1982, also adopt a broad-brush approach. Yet although everyone must fulfil the requirements, the content and quality of each experience varies enormously from one school to another. The skeleton syllabuses are proposed as models by the statutory bodies, but the reality depends on the tutors, the clinical settings, the number of students and so on. The statutory bodies, perhaps because they could do little without more money for ward staff and teachers, seem to have adopted a rather laissez-faire approach, constrained also by the need to produce a certain number of new nurses every year to take the places of the large numbers who leave. The new approaches outlined in the syllabuses also make bigger demands on the tutors, who may be ill-equipped to cope through lack of training in new teaching methods, and may lack the time, resources or motivation to update themselves.

In some respects the content of nurse education is most remarkable for what it leaves out. Much of nursing care involves working with people who are suffering, mentally or physically, yet general training fails to equip us to deal with this. It does not help us to know what to say when people ask difficult questions, and it does not help us as individuals to cope with the distress or fear experienced due to constant closeness to others' suffering. Psychiatric nurses obviously have more training and support of this kind, but they too go through the same kind of stress — which produces the symptoms of exhaustion and apathy described as 'burn-out' and forces many people to leave. It is also being recognised that nursing care which is individualised and patient-centred can create a more intense relationship between nurse and patient, and that caring for the whole person means the nurse needs plenty of support too.

The prevailing attitude is that if we ignore the pain it will simply go away. Nurses are not supposed to show their feelings; crying when a patient dies is getting 'too' involved and is frowned on as unprofessional. Equally there is pressure to get on with all the patients, and no attempt is made to talk about the anger or resentment which nurses feel towards particular patients — even though psychiatry acknowledges that releasing feelings and dealing with them openly and with the support of colleagues and friends is much healthier for all concerned.

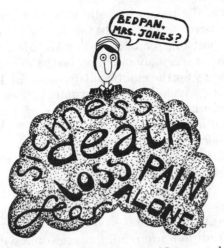

Patients' feelings are denied too. Nurses who have not learned to come to terms with their own fear or anger are not well placed to support their patients, and studies have shown how anyone who does not conform to the cheerful, compliant ideal is labelled as a 'difficult' patient — when they are the ones often most in need of help. This refusal to acknowledge patients' feelings is not based on cruelty, but on an inability to cope with them — which brings us back to the lack of preparation in school and on the ward. 'Reassure the patient', we are told over and over again — but reassure them of what? That they will be all right, when we know they are dying? That it won't hurt, when the chances are that it will? By pretending the problems don't exist, it's not the patients we are trying to reassure, but ourselves.

Nearly 25 years ago sociologist Isobel Menzies documented the way hospital routine is organised to protect the staff from psychological trauma. Her work, *A Case Study in the Functioning of Social Systems as a Defence against Anxiety*, underlines the point that nursing 'whole patients' rather than completing a series of tasks may create big emotional problems which in many ways the old system was designed, at least unconsciously, to avoid. Whisking round the ward taking all the temperatures or doing the 'back round', the nurse develops a protective armour to avoid the complex demands of 30 patients, and always has the excuse of having to move on to the next when she gets into deep water, an escape route perhaps less easily taken when she is responsible for only half a dozen or less. Yet Menzies' observations have never been seriously taken on board to prepare nurses more adequately for the emotional demands of the job and to understand the psychological interactions. Few other occupations could match the baptism of fire of, say, sending a new student nurse to lay out the corpse of a patient she has nursed and become fond of, with no preparation or follow-up, and then telling her to 'pull herself together' when she is found crying in the sluice.

All these criticisms have been aired in canteens, conferences and journals, but the slowness of the response is immensely frustrating. In a system notable for its rigidity and love of tradition, innovation is regarded with suspicion and there is a fear of failure which discourages experimentation. Perhaps the new statutory bodies will have a galvanising effect, but whatever they do they will need support from a government prepared to invest in nursing education — for the sake of future health care — instead of cutting resources while uttering platitudes about dedication and service.

Teaching methods

'Nursing has not been able to use accepted educational methods such as reasoning from first principles and working from the known to the unknown', writes Monica Baly in *Nursing and Social Change*. 'Techniques had to be performed and jobs done by the person on hand to do them, and if there was time to show "how" there was seldom time to explain "why". The service needs took precedence over the educational needs of the student.' Substituting the present tense for Baly's past tense gives us a reasonable description of the state of nursing education today and the poor quality of its methods. It applies not only to the school, but to the clinical learning environments on the ward and in the community.

The gap between theory and practice in nursing education is universally recognised as a major problem. It is agreed that on-the-job learning, backed up by private study and short periods of classroom work, is the best approach for a practical discipline like nursing, and research shows that students learn more readily in the clinical setting. Nonetheless the foundation is laid in the school, where notes are taken on specific procedures or the nursing care of patients with a particular disease and the student refers to them for her exam revision. Everyone is shocked to find that things aren't done that way on the ward — sometimes because the tutor has failed to keep pace with changes in daily practice, but more often because in the rush to finish the work, corners are cut and routines are not adhered to. The heavy ward workload means that qualified staff — even those with a strong commitment to teach, which not all share — may find it hard to tear themselves away from the routine and to spend time working with students or holding more formal teaching sessions. The trend is now to emphasise the teaching responsibilities of trained nurses, but few are equipped to carry that burden. Ward-based formal teaching can be nerve-racking for those who have little or no preparation for it, like most staff nurses and sisters, and the pressure of work is always a handy excuse to avoid it. Working one-to-one with a student is avoided by the nurse who lacks both time and confidence.

Instead students tend to learn not so much from qualified staff as from other students or auxiliaries — so what they pick up is often incomplete, wrong or reliant on unthinking routine. With a lack of staff or equipment, people soon learn how to cut corners in their anxiety to finish 'on time' or else risk a reprimand, which lays a poor foundation for later practice as well as giving patients inferior quality care or even putting them at risk. Bad habits and incorrect procedures are passed on unwittingly from one student to another.

Related to this unsatisfactory way of picking up the rudiments of the job is the tendency to cover up mistakes and ignorance. The pressure to appear efficient and capable makes it difficult for any nurse to admit to not knowing something, or to discuss whether there might be a better approach to a particular problem or procedure. This is shown in the expectations of what students should be able to do at each stage in training. When a senior nurse says, 'You're a third year — you know how to insert a catheter, don't you,' the student must be very sure of herself to confess that she doesn't know and to risk being scorned, even though there is no reason why she 'should' know how to pass a urinary catheter if she has never seen it done or had the opportunity to do it under supervision. Such an attitude also assumes there is a set way to do things, and implies teaching by rote rather than by principle.

The problems of ward-based teaching are not helped by the frequent lack of contact between school and hospital. The grade of clinical teacher was introduced specifically to take some of the teaching load off ward staff, and to help bridge the gap, but staff shortages and personal insecurities mean clinical teachers are rarely seen in many places, especially at night when they could have more scope to work with students. The insecurity of ward staff often leads them to see the clinical teacher as a threat to their authority rather than a helpful colleague; they fear she will criticise and undermine them. There is a standing joke that clinical teachers take hours to do simple bed-baths — meaning they are too fussy and are not aware of the pressure of work. The teachers, for their part, feel out of place and short on clinical credibility and have no power to do anything about bad practice they see on the wards, other than trying to teach their own students in the small time available.

Learning in school also has its drawbacks. The drastic shortage of nurse teachers means classes are often huge — 40 students or more — which tempts them into presenting the material in indigestible lecture form rather than adopting more exploratory and exciting methods such as work in small groups. Tutors who have so many students in their charge also find it more difficult to develop the close student-teacher relationships which encourage an open and supportive approach with space for each person to grow.

Instead, the weeks in school often become a mindless gallop through an uninspiring syllabus, scribbling notes through hours of boring classes in the knowledge that these facts will later have to be regurgitated in an exam. Audiovisual aids such as video and tape-slide shows help to liven things up, but they are not properly used. One ward sister recently devised a tape-slide programme on the care of the elderly, which she sent out with explicit instructions about how it should only be used in the framework of group discussion, and found it was being played straight through with no conversation at all, while the tutors disappeared to mark another set of essays. Basic nursing education is seen not as the beginning of a life-long learning process, but as a finite period in which a specified amount of information must be crammed into the student's head. Often this knowledge is not taught from principles; there is little attempt to encourage skills which can be employed in self-directed learning, and little opportunity or enthusiasm to use more imaginative forms of learning such as role-play.

These shortcomings are bolstered by a system in which passing an exam rather than improving your practice is seen as the main goal. Proof of ability to present written material coherently, and to demonstrate knowledge of certain facts, is no bad thing, but from Nightingale onwards many people have complained that written exams are an inappropriate test of nursing skills. So the final exams are supplemented by practical assessments and records of progress. There are still many protests that good nurses fail and bad ones pass. Any exam system produces odd results, but the biggest danger is the way such a system shapes attitudes to education.

The student nurse is pulled in two directions by the demands of the service and her own educational needs. Low pay, authoritarian discipline and demeaning treatment are justified by the excuse that she is only a trainee and must earn the right to be treated decently ('what was good enough for us is good enough for you'). Individuality is denied and nursing students are treated as pairs of hands; personal problems and individual learning difficulties are ignored. There is pious talk of the profession's future lying in students' hands, but that future is jeopardised every day when emotional and educational needs are submerged in the struggle to get the work done or to scrape through an exam.

The student is also caught in the crossfire of an old hostility between senior nurses in education and service. Service managers resent any implication that standards are not up to scratch, regarding tutors as ivory-tower theorists, while educationalists are forgetful of the enormous difficulty of running services and providing ward-based teaching on a shoestring. Relations can be so bad that in one school of nursing the director of nursing education was never known to set foot in the hospital a hundred yards from her door — hardly an atmosphere for encouraging the cooperation necessary to develop good educational programmes.

One way in which senior nurses collude in exploiting students is in the abuse or manipulation of official training requirements. The training bodies stipulate the time to be spent in each specialty, and also lay down minimum experiences in night duty. Yet most students are unaware that they only have to do 24 weeks on nights to fulfil the requirement, and most work much more, often with minimal staffing and little support from qualified staff. Allocation officers are known to declare that 'it's in the rules', but no-one is *asked* if they are prepared to work extra nights because the service needs them — or else they are asked in a way which admits no refusal. The good nurse does what she's told.

Students are also told to do split shifts or relief work to help out, regardless of its educational value. They have little power to object, but at least knowing the ground rules will make it clear if a hospital/school is consistently exploiting its learners. Protests may then be made to put pressure on for better staffing, and it is the responsibility of senior staff to see that those protests are taken up to the highest levels. After all, training approval can be withdrawn for persistent exploitation — which would force the hospital to reconsider its ways.

Finding out what the rules are is no mean feat in itself. Hitherto they have been published as circulars sent to all schools and authorities, but not to individual nurses; they are often updated in new documents, and difficult to track down. Some of the rules are quite complicated and badly expressed, and all vary according to the type and length of training being undertaken. Some enlightened places are now issuing new recruits with a folder of information covering rules, sickness, employment law and so on, an example all should follow; the statutory bodies, in fact, could insist on it.

Time for a change

Looking at nursing education, it is easy to fall into the trap of reproducing the existing hierarchy of status and priority. In particular it is tempting to concentrate on hospital nursing — much of our training being hospital-based — and on acute medical and surgical nursing at that, rather than the care of the elderly and other long-stay patients, or community services. We are so used to seeing the acute hospital as the focus of modern health care that it is hard to take a fresh look at what kind of care and what setting will meet future needs, or even to ask ourselves whether nursing itself is the most suitable discipline in which to develop some new approaches, since it is so rooted in particular traditions.

Sometimes the problems of the present — and there are many of them — inhibit a broader view of today, let alone tomorrow. Even a cursory look at the state of the NHS reveals facts which nursing practice and education fail to take into account. Perhaps the most surprising, and contrary to the bias of our training, is that around half the hospital beds in the UK are occupied by long-stay patients, mainly the elderly, the mentally handicapped and the mentally ill. Far less money is spent on each long-stay resident than on each patient in an acute hospital, although the hospital is often their only home — and this includes not only money spent on medical attention, which you might expect to be less, but on laundry, meals and cleaning as well as nursing. Nursing costs, which you might expect to be similar, are far lower per patient because there are larger numbers of cheaper untrained staff, and fewer nurses for each patient, even though the care given is almost exclusively nursing care.

In fact most people's contact with the NHS does not occur through hospitals but through community-based services such as birth control clinics and general practices. Women are the most frequent users, visiting clinics for contraception, antenatal care and child health, while elderly and disabled people often use community nursing services. Health visitors offer a preventive service promoting good health, and psychiatric nurses are beginning to work with people in their own homes. Although acute hospitals have the lion's share of power, status and resources, most people's experience of health care takes place outside hospitals.

The pressure on community services increases daily. The proportion of elderly people in the population, who inevitably make extensive use of the NHS because of the problems of ageing, is rising, while better standards of housing and diet and modern medical techniques improve the survival chances of people, born handicapped or falling ill, who may require long-term support. Changing circumstances make it hard to measure whether people are using health services more, but factors such as the isolation of urban life and the acceptance of the right to welfare probably encourage more frequent visits to the GP and use of nursing services. Cuts in the NHS budget and early discharge policies are also shifting a bigger workload on to community staff, who are not receiving extra support to cope with it. The closure of many small hospitals, begun by the Labour government in 1974–9 and accelerated by the Conservatives, has led to a quicker turnover of patients in the remaining acute hospitals (industrial terms like 'turnover' and 'throughput' are increasingly being used by managers, as though the NHS were a business). While it is agreed that in some circumstances patients do better at home and prefer earlier discharge, the great pressure on beds and the enormous waiting lists mean people are often going home before they can really look after themselves — with community staff and relatives taking the strain.

Yet while the community services continue to be poorly funded, governments of both colours are blithely discussing moving care 'into the community'. Everyone agrees that most people who are mentally ill, mentally handicapped, old or the social outcasts of the past should not have to live out their lives in large, impersonal, isolated and often depressing long-stay hospitals — but the politicians are not prepared to back up their promises with cash, nor are they prepared to take on the powerful acute hospital consultants to ensure that NHS money is distributed more fairly. Mentally handicapped people still live in rows of beds six inches apart, while consultants use NHS money to buy scanners and keep dying people alive with expensive experimental drugs.

In some places the old institutions are being closed and the revenue used to run small, comfortable homes for the residents, though sometimes the money gained from such closures seems to vanish without trace. More staff will be needed to implement the new policies, for a higher nurse-patient ratio is needed — a small home cannot get by with two nurses to 40 residents. But the move will be disastrous if nurses now in hospitals are simply uprooted and put to work in hostels. Their training, based in hospital, does not equip them well to work in a different setting, any more than hospital-based training equips general nurses to work on the district (acknowledged in the fact that district nurse training is now mandatory for practice). Traditional hospital training churns out plenty of nurses who can dole out tranquillisers or handle machines, but not so many who can teach a stroke patient to move from bed to chair or help someone deal with a drink problem in their own home.

If nursing training were changed overnight to match changing health needs, instead of conforming to outdated medical ideas, it would probably be almost unrecognisable. It would not emphasise pathology, but would start with health; it would be geared to encouraging independence, not submission, in both nurses and patients. It would concentrate on meeting the needs of daily living, not on the requirements of doctors; and it would not be based so exclusively in hospitals.

The new statutory bodies

Such changes might at last be possible in nursing education with the arrival of the new statutory bodies, which are legally responsible for the training and conduct of nurses and midwives. The 1979 Nurses, Midwives and Health Visitors Act has given the UK Central Council and national boards more sweeping powers than any previous body, including the prospect of controlling the nurse education budget, currently split between statutory bodies and health authorities. They have already produced a stream of documents on education, professional conduct, the new single professional register and so on, but is there any evidence that they will push forward the much-needed radical overhaul?

It is early days, but judging by the output to date there is not much to suggest that the bodies see the problems outlined above as a priority, or contain the necessary strategic outlook and skills. Much discussion has focussed on matters of professional and national rivalry as different groups and the four national boards assert their independence. Such wrangling may be a necessary staking out of ground before the policy arguments begin in earnest, but it is worrying that the documents themselves concentrate on matters internal to nursing, such as the structure (but not the content) of training rather than the health needs of the UK. They start at the wrong end, with the nurse and not the patient, with professional demands rather than users' needs.

Is it actually open to any statutory body to approach its responsibilities in such a radical way? Few others have had the courage to do so. But if our first duty really is to the public, and if we really care more about health than about our own professional rivalries, then the new bodies will have the support to carve out for themselves an innovatory role as defenders of the ill and underprivileged rather than as maintainers of the status quo.

Educationally, perhaps the most important idea which has emerged in the UKCC consultation papers is the belief that registration should be the beginning and not the end of a nurse's training. Linked with the need to prepare qualified staff for their new posts, and with the introduction of a requirement that every nurse must prove her entitlement to practise when applying for a periodic licence, this notion of 'continuing education' is becoming very popular, though it too demands big, and unlikely, increases in staff and resources, as well as changes in attitude. The qualified nurse, they say, should keep up to date and continue to broaden and deepen her knowledge through clinical courses, management training, seminars, private study and so on. But not only does time mean money; many nurses have a strong anti-education bias. Introducing a statutory requirement of proving entitlement to practise has been done long since by midwives, whose proof of fitness to continue in practice usually consists of attendance at a refresher course. Keeping the requirements as flexible as possible will enable them to be tailored to individual preferences, and a statutory requirement might also prove a useful lever in the battle for resources.

Further Reading

Baly M. (1980). *Nursing and Social Change.* 2nd edn. London: William Heinemann Medical Books.

Beardshaw V. (1981). *Conscientious Objectors at Work.* London: Social Audit.

Dickinson S. (1982). The Nursing Process and the Professional Status of Nursing. *Nursing Times,* Occasional Paper; June 2.

Doyal L. (1980). *The Political Economy of Health.* London: Pluto Press.

Melia K. (1983). Students' Views of Nursing, series in *Nursing Times*: Discussion of Method and Just Passing Through, May 18, pp. 24–7; Nursing in the Dark, May 25, pp. 62–3; Doing Nursing and Being Professional, June 1, pp. 28–30.

Menzies I. (1960). *A Case Study in the Functioning of Social Systems as a Defence Against Anxiety.* London: Tavistock.

Nurses, Midwives and Health Visitors Act (1979). London: HMSO.

Nurses, Midwives and Health Visitors Rules Approval Order No. 873 (1983). London: HMSO.

Report of the Committee on Nursing (Briggs Report; 1972). London: HMSO.

UKCC. (1982 and onwards). Consultation papers from working groups, especially Working Group 3 on education and training, and Working Group 2 on the single professional register.

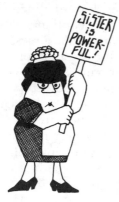

4

Into
the profession

The formal content of nursing education, on the wards and in school, is an essential part of the preparation to be a qualified nurse. But nursing is also a complex and long-established social system in which 'tradition', 'discipline', 'hierarchy' and 'profession' are elements which may be just as important in producing the ideal nurse as defined by that system. It attempts to reproduce its values in its recruits, who are often poorly equipped to challenge them or even to realise what is happening to them.

At least half of all nursing students are school-leavers, usually living away from home for the first time and so particularly susceptible to an institution whose values seem to offer comfort and security. Lacking confidence and wide experience, they may find it hard publicly to question the assumptions and ideologies they are introduced to, especially when these are presented by senior staff who — for good or ill — have considerable power over them. Strict discipline, the fear of victimisation, lack of knowledge about rights, the tutor's power to require extra classroom work and the sister's authority to refuse off-duty requests all help to instil the desired attitudes in students, whether they are conscious of them or not.

The values which the student encounters in the school of nursing and on the wards are found at all levels of the nursing hierarchy. The professional and statutory bodies are gradually shaking off the twin set and pearls image, but conferences and nursing journals still reveal a strong interest in status, titles, New Year honours and royal visits. A major event in the nursing calendar is Florence Nightingale's birthday, when coachloads of impeccably uniformed nurses are shipped off to Westminster Abbey for a commemoration service which includes matron carrying the notorious lamp down the aisle. This traditionalism, and not the hurly-burly of NHS management at a high level, is the image of their seniors absorbed by junior nurses. Early pep-talks from the director of nurse education or district nursing officer are more likely to appeal to a sense of tradition and loyalty to a hierarchy and a profession than to look at the reality of nursing work.

Many influences can be traced in the 'socialisation' of a nurse, a process which imbues her with a set of values and expectations designed to ensure she takes her place in the system and thereby helps to keep it going on the same lines. Even before she becomes a student, part of that process has already taken place through gender expectations about the nature of the nurse and her work, which affect both men and women in nursing. As soon as she starts training, she is also subjected to the powerful influence of the nursing hierarchy and its notion of professionalism in nursing.

The hierarchy

The structure of the nursing workforce is most easily likened to a pyramid. Right at the bottom, or base, are the most numerous grades, nursing auxiliaries and assistants, with the students just above them. Then there are enrolled nurses, sisters, nursing officers and so on up to the regional nursing officers at the top (with, perhaps, the Civil Service's four chief nursing officers above them). Over the past 20 years there have been many confusing changes in the titles of various grades, owing to NHS and internal nursing reorgan- isations, but the essential shape has barely altered. Service and management grades are contained in the same structure, although the education hierarchy perhaps needs a smaller pyramid of its own; it occupies a rather ambiguous space somewhere between the service and the statutory bodies.

The pyramid structure of authority is familiar in our society and therefore appears 'natural', though its relevance to nursing care is now being questioned. Authority is vested from above in those lower down, with wages, as well as power over others, rising as you move higher up. Yet the higher up you are, the more removed you are from direct contact with patients — supposedly the reason for nursing's existence. Caring for patients is always said to be the nurse's priority, yet those who move up and away from direct contact ironically get greater rewards in money, status and authority. What value is really placed on care by such a system — which leaves the patients for most of the time in the hands of those with the least experience or education, the students and auxiliaries?

From the bottom looking up, the main impression is of large numbers of unseen senior people issuing orders which are passed down the line — paralleled by the frequently encountered inability of anyone in the structure to make a decision without referring to someone higher up, although again those at the bottom are making crucial nursing decisions all the time. The people at the bottom have little contact with those above sister grade, on the whole, and when they do it tends to be a negative experience; even going to the nursing office to report back after sick leave feels like confessing a crime. Junior nurses are used to meeting indifference or even hostility, rather than warmth and interest.

The hierarchical structure has been justified on the grounds that it is necessary for a clear allocation of responsibility and control over other staff. There are indeed some situations in which someone should take charge and direct others (usually emergencies), but unfortunately there are countless more situations in which the power is exercised for its own sake or to conceal insecurities. Occupying a defined place in a hierarchy is comforting, and always offers the opportunity for decisions to be passed on to someone else, but the hierarchical structure does not usually serve the best interests of either patients or nurses.

Everyone in nursing has at some time experienced the abuse of power by someone more senior, and has been hurt by it, yet the system is difficult to modify. Our training does little to make us into strong and independent people who can make decisions based on cool assessments, or who are happy to be responsible for the consequences of any decisions. Almost inevitably when we are given the positions of authority for which we are so ill prepared, it is tempting to cling to the trappings of titles, uniforms and privileges. Students start by being discouraged from expressing their doubts and fears, and continue by converting them to misdirected anger or bullying — of patients and other staff — in order to appear so certain and authoritative that no-one will dare question them.

The strength of tradition in nursing may be a key to the continuing survival of this increasingly outdated and unhelpful structure. A hierarchy prescribes certain ways of behaving and occupying its grades, and gives power to people who, outside that system, might be powerless. The more independent and self-supporting people are, the less they need to rely on a fixed order or the support of a predefined role. In nursing such people tend to work in the community or develop their own specialty (in stoma care, say, or behavioural therapy) which gives them the independence they desire. But on the whole nurses tend to lack such independence, because of their gender, class, low status and socialisation, and most attempts to break through this are unsupported or deliberately blocked.

The hierarchical organisation of nursing has all sorts of disadvantages for those low down, who have to bear the brunt of more senior nurses passing the buck, refusing to be responsible for their actions and giving the unpleasant jobs to those below them (so the staff nurse does the 'essential' paperwork while the student is sent off to do a rectal washout). But the relationship is also extended to areas which have nothing to do with work and should be private. Some senior nurses criticise the appearance or behaviour of juniors off duty, which can be upsetting and insulting — especially when the nurse is living in hospital accommodation and may find it hard to escape this kind of surveillance and invasion of privacy. The sister who marches unannounced into a student's room to 'check up' on her when she is off sick is just one familiar example of the many infringements of nurses' privacy and personal integrity. Yet most people say nothing because the consequences of objecting, they feel, would be even worse.

Many of the stories of nurse's inhumanity to nurse are hardly believed when told to friends outside the job, yet are all too familiar inside it. The student nurse forced to return to a late shift after her father's funeral, the nurse whose unwanted pregnancy was reported to the school in breach of confidence, the enrolled nurse awoken at midday after night duty with a non-urgent query about a drip are not exceptional incidents but common occurrences.

What happens to senior nurses to turn them into such monsters — or is it just that people are more likely to remember and relate the hostile and upsetting incidents than the acts of kindness? Antipathy for 'the boss' is common in most jobs, for the manager seems to have a cushy life protected from the grubby exhaustion of the ward or production line. To some extent dislike of senior nurses as people in authority is hardly unexpected, yet the vigour with which many nurses express their hostility — including senior nurses themselves remembering their own experiences as juniors — suggests some deeper malaise beyond the normal pattern.

The discussion provoked by the government's implementation of the Griffiths management inquiry recommendations has brought to the fore this gap between nurse managers and the rest. Amid the exhortations to stand shoulder to shoulder and defend the profession, there have been widespread criticisms of nurse management, with many nurses feeling they would be no worse, or even better off being managed by someone who was not a nurse. Some criticism of the performance of nurse managers is deserved, yet a part of the hostility has more to do with this unspecified

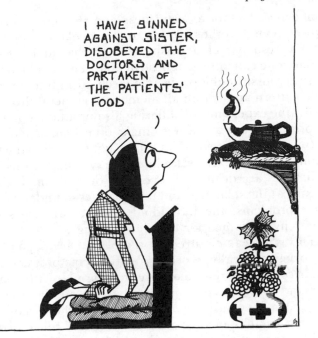

and unexplored antipathy, much of it probably stemming from those early experiences.

That feeling often spills over into emotional attacks on nurse management, in which those lower down the hierarchy declare that the managers do nothing, are unnecessary, make life difficult and so on. It is important to analyse these attacks because they express something which lies close to the heart of the nursing experience. Also, by the force of their emotional appeal, they make it more difficult to hold a sensible debate about the undoubted need to manage a service involving so many people, so much equipment and so much money.

Many senior nurses behave in such a heartless and insulting way to juniors that it is hard to believe they have been through similar experiences themselves. But therein perhaps lies the key; the experience of becoming a nurse and rising through the ranks leaves so many scars that self-protection is the only route most people can follow. Insecurity, lack of confidence, lack of assertiveness and the often unrealistic expectations of other people may provoke a very natural human response of defensiveness, so that at least on the surface one can appear indestructible. Years of behaving in this way fossilise the protective mechanism into an immutable pattern and cut off all memory of vulnerability. Often, sadly, the experience of suffering also produces not a desire to prevent it but an urge to make others suffer too.

It is absolutely crucial for nurses not to fall into the trap of blaming individuals for faults in the system, yet this is how difficulties are dealt with over and over again. Instead of looking at the structure and its dynamics to understand and solve problems, the individual nurse at all levels of the hierarchy is blamed for her shortcomings.

This is a bleak picture, but there are a few hopeful signs. In society generally, working relationships between people are becoming more relaxed and less formal, with consultation and consensus decisions probably more the norm than they have previously been. Like many other occupations, nursing has loosened up and become less concerned with rigid structures and relationships and 'knowing your place'. It is more widely accepted that a nurse's personal life is her own affair, and also that many nurses have families and partnerships which demand some of her time and attention — she is not expected to be a martyr to her job quite so often.

More specifically, many nurses believe that the old-style hierarchy no longer meets the needs of nurses or patients. It is acknowledged that patients want and should be able to participate in planning and carrying out their care and treatment, and with growing pressure from consumer groups and individuals, the health care professions are having to rethink their old assumptions about being in charge and telling the patient what is best for him or her. It is also becoming clear that in many ways patients are more likely to cope better with their illness or disability if they are in partnership with health workers, rather than under their thumbs.

The moves afoot to develop a new career structure for clinical nurses, and indeed to take a fresh look at the entire hierarchy, are partly a response to these changes, although they have other causes too. By stating a belief that each qualified nurse should be a practitioner in her own right and that, prepared by good education (rather than training), she should relate to other nurses not as seniors or juniors but as colleagues engaged in the same work and sharing the same goals, the new thinking is offering a way out of hidebound tradition and hierarchy.

Nursing auxiliaries

Often the senior nurses who cling most firmly to the idea of hierarchy and find most security in it are the same people who espouse the cause of professionalism, or else already believe that nursing has attained professional status. They do not see the contradiction in their position; a true professional who is an independent practitioner accountable to patients and peers for her practice has no need of any army-style structure to keep her in line. They also have problems in reconciling the contradiction inherent in being part of an occupational group whose base, in the pyramid structure, is thousands and thousands of unqualified staff — a quarter of the nursing workforce as defined by the DHSS. Where you stand in the professionalism debate depends largely on your attitude to these colleagues.

Much nursing, and most of the direct patient care, is carried out not by qualified nurses but by nursing auxiliaries (called nursing assistants in mental illness and mental handicap hospitals). This distresses some of the nursing leaders, and the issue causes much bitterness. Is it right that people should be looked after by untrained staff? Is the nursing care which auxiliaries give inferior?

Recently the RCN has been talking about having a 'professional nursing service', i.e. consisting entirely of trained nurses and those in training, by the end of the century. Even if the college's belief that this would mean higher standards of nursing care is correct, the chances of it happening are remote. In some areas, mental handicap for example, the ratio of untrained to trained staff is actually increasing, while cuts in budgets encourage authorities to employ the cheapest staff available, such as nursing auxiliaries. What is remarkable about the attitudes of the RCN and other professional and statutory bodies is that the reality of who staffs the wards is barely acknowledged, let alone fully discussed. The plans to develop a new career structure say very little about the role of untrained staff, and yet it is untrained staff who will continue to give the bulk of the bedside care.

This ostrich syndrome partly stems from the nursing leaders' enormous desire to establish nursing as a profession. It is almost as though their need to insist that good nursing is synonymous with good preparation (the importance of training and qualification) blindfolds them to the facts of what happens in most hospitals — or perhaps it is because most of them, by virtue of their senior positions, rarely set foot on a ward or in a patient's home. Understanding the urge to win recognition of nursing as a profession is crucial to any understanding of nursing today and will be talked about in more detail, but it is worth noting here in the context of untrained staff — because establishing nurses as an elite group of highly skilled people who deserve more money, status and power depends on limiting their numbers. Doctors, administrators and the public will hardly grant that recognition and its accompanying demands when there are thousands of people doing the job who lack academic or professional qualifications. The RCN and those of like minds still want to retain firm managerial control of untrained staff, but their strategy depends on segregating auxiliaries from the rest and putting them at a distance. It is no coincidence that the RCN fought hard to have auxiliaries excluded from the pay review body and managed to extract some 'concessions' from the government on the issue.

Nursing auxiliaries are a neglected group of people, not least by their own fellow workers, and in the long run, ironically, their needs might be best served by a clear separation from qualified nurses, though it is doubtful whether this would benefit patients. The nursing hierarchy has not lifted a finger to help auxiliaries, even though they are appallingly badly paid, often have to do two jobs if they are looking after

'For six months I worked part-time as a nursing auxiliary on a men's surgical ward. When I left, the sister said, "I bet you've hated every minute of it, haven't you?" In fact I had surprised myself by caring so much about the "routine" work of bed-baths, feeding, helping, talking. It was absolutely basic, all of it necessary and all of it capable of transforming for better or worse the quality of someone's existence at a time when he or she is vulnerable and (often embarrassingly) dependent. What outraged me were the assumptions about me which seemed to be shared by most of the staff "above" the level of ward sister, and by a number of them "below" and at that level, but rarely by patients and never by ancillary workers. Assumptions that an auxiliary has an amazingly strong body, a mind limited to "small talk", and a name you needn't remember . . . and that if one or all of these elements were missing, then by definition she would be unhappy in her work.

A number of things disturbed me deeply. At the worst time possible, hospital rules cut us off from people who were dying, forced us to play games of pretending they would get better, to manipulate our conversations on to things which had less and less meaning, or even to avoid spending time with them so as not to be confronted with a straight question or a request to talk about their approaching death. The basic pattern of work involved doing things for or to the patients rather than being with them, talking, sharing their experiences. Orderlies and cleaners related to the patients as people most of the time, but as an auxiliary I felt caught between their way of working and "the nurse's role", which involved reducing people to patients whose dignity could be sacrificed to the procedures of nursing care. It's a shame that, as with orderlies and cleaners, and often nurses too, much of the skilled human rather than technical care that I could have offered was neither expected nor allowed.'

A former nursing auxiliary, Liverpool

children and a home, often have the most unpleasant and unrewarding tasks, often work part-time and miss out on work and union benefits, and often suffer from racism too as many of them are black. There has been virtually no serious, extended discussion of the role auxiliaries play in caring for patients, despite its importance, with one or two notable exceptions. Auxiliaries are condemned for their ignorance but resented if they try to learn, while their acquired knowledge is ignored or dismissed. Nurses often talk about caring, but the lack of consideration given to their own colleagues is shameful.

Some authorities provide in-service (on the job) training for auxiliaries, but it is rarely more than the odd day or two. The RCN has recently opposed the introduction of a national training programme, while unions like COHSE and NUPE, whose nursing membership is hugely swelled by auxiliaries, do not regard them as a very high priority, although this is changing. Some of the most positive thinking about preparing untrained people for nursing work — which will increase their satisfaction as well as improve care — is coming from charities like Help the Aged. As it pointed out in 1982, 'their title and job description imply that their work is to help trained nurses, but inevitably they are expected to carry out a range of nursing procedures, often without close supervision.'

Help the Aged has produced a training pack for auxiliaries who work with old people. This was described by the RCN as 'a useful adjunct in the basic instruction of nursing auxiliaries', a revealing phrase — why is education regarded as the goal for professional nurses while 'instruction' is good enough for auxiliaries? The pack looks at topics such as incontinence, 'difficult' patients, death, and the importance of choice to people living in institutions, discussing them in a simple but sensitive way and affirming an awareness that untrained staff are incredibly important in many patients' lives. The fact that such work was done outside the nursing or even NHS establishment is yet another illustration of their poor record in this field.

'Nurses' preoccupation with routine may mean we fail to see that another way of doing things could be an improvement, so changes are very slowly made and accepted. Thus the nurse may become the slave of routine. Linked with this is the attitude of deference to medical staff and to all senior nursing staff. This deference goes beyond what is called for by the system of line management. It is built in from an early stage by such actions as that of the doctor or charge nurse who, on a ward round of the patients, comes inside the screens while you are bed-bathing a patient and expects you immediately to leave or to fade into the background. The patient is expected to join in with this deferential attitude, and not to mind this invasion of his privacy; he waits quietly while the professionals talk about him over his head, as a case, and speaks only when spoken to. This habitual deference may largely be responsible for nurses' reluctance to speak out for what we feel is right or needs changing. We are often afraid to take a stand against those above us in the hierarchy.'

Student nurse, London

Profession, craft or just a job?

'Profession', 'professional' and 'professionalism' are words which nurses often hear. Journals and textbooks are peppered with them and tutors and sisters are prone to use them, often as terms of approval: 'professional' behaviour is supposed to be the right way to behave, a professional nurse is a good nurse, our occupation is described as a profession.

Partly this is a reflection of the current popularity of the word, as in the phrases 'professional musician' or 'professional footballer' (who even commits professional fouls). It implies payment for special skills, in contrast to the amateur, and it also implies proficiency and concentration on the task in hand. Beyond this popular use, though, nursing seems to be obsessed with the idea — the attempt to establish our occupation as a profession has been the single most important concern of nursing leaders in recent years. There are many arguments for and against this strategy of trying to win recognition as a profession, often voiced in the journals and at conferences. These may seem rather irrelevant to the nurse on the ward or in the community, but at the same time they undoubtedly strike some chord with many; it is important to sort out what is implied in the value-laden approval of professionalism.

The current preoccupation with the professional status of nursing has largely ousted the idea of nursing as a vocation, which is now seen as rather outdated, though it tends to be dusted off in particular disputes such as those over pay. In fact the arguments about profession v. vocation began a century ago or more; Nightingale commented, '*they* call it a profession, but I say that it is a calling.' For her it was tied up with a belief that she was performing a mission from God. Religious commitment is still an important motive for many entering nursing, and there are many fruitful comparisons to be made between nursing and a religious calling. The new idea of professionalism, however, attempts to embrace the dedication to work and set of high ideals which is implied in a vocation, while discarding the submissive attributes; it also contains implied changes in the social status of ill people and their relationships with health workers.

Above all the word 'profession', unlike 'vocation' or 'calling', seems to suggest independence, autonomy and control over your own work. Many nurses resent their subservience to doctors, while others who are less bothered still welcome the idea of better social status which the word implies. Being a member of a profession is much grander than simply doing a job, and of course all nurses work alongside a superb example of a professional, the doctor. Doctors have money, high social standing and autonomy, so why shouldn't we, think many nurses. Their power to control their own work and to make decisions is enviable and is brought home to nurses every day. A patient's medication needs to be changed and the nurse may know exactly what he or she needs, but she must await the medical signature, even for an aspirin. Admittedly such power also carries great responsibility, yet nurses themselves bear similar burdens but lack both the power to discharge those duties fully, and the substantial material rewards and fringe benefits.

The medical profession has many attributes which nurses would like to possess themselves. In the public mind health care and medicine are mistakenly equated, and doctors are extremely powerful in influencing policy and deciding how NHS money is spent, even in areas about which they know comparatively little. Nurses know that good nursing is just as important to the patient's welfare as good doctoring, but this is not reflected in the relative amounts spent on training nurses and doctors, in medical and nursing research, in fees paid to medical and nursing lecturers, in time off for study, in salaries, and in many other things. Nurses may injure their backs through a lack of lifting equipment while doctors can successfully claim money for expensive technical machinery of doubtful therapeutic value. When it comes to cutting the NHS cake, the need for adequate nursing staff levels may be more crucial than the need for a new specialist unit or a scanner, but almost invariably 'medical need' or 'clinical judgement', in other words doctors' preferences, win the argument.

The desire for greater autonomy, which nurses tend to equate with a desire to enjoy the same advantages as doctors, is often linked with the desire to improve standards of care. This assumption that professionalism means excellence is often used to justify the professions' positions of superiority; they say they are protecting the public by controlling the recruitment and training of people who want to join them. On the whole nurses appear to have accepted very uncritically the professions' description of their function as protectors of the public; they have not examined the negative aspects of professionalism and the greed and elitism with which it is often associated. Unfortunately the genuine urge to improve health care has become mixed up with other difficult arguments and uncomfortable or undesirable implications, to the point where nurses who say they oppose using professionalism as a strategy to improve care are not given a serious hearing.

A critical look at the record of occupations usually defined as true professions — such as medicine and the law — reveals some worrying facts. For example, the reasons for restricting entry to the profession often seem to spring not so much from concern for public welfare as from a desire to stop others muscling in on a profitable job. Limiting the availability of a doctor or a lawyer enables each to charge more for his services and to establish a monopoly. Midwifery is a prime example: 19th century doctors became concerned about obstetric care not only from a desire to help mothers, but from a desire to take control of this potentially profitable and prestigious area. Instead of helping to improve the midwives' care, they attempted to exclude them from practice, with some success. So today midwives are having to fight for recognition of their role as the key worker in normal childbirth, a position they occupied long before obstetricians came on the scene.

Being a profession, then, has a variety of implications, and not all of them are desirable ones. Nurses should not go along with the assumption that winning professional status for nursing would mean nothing but good for nurses and patients. In any case it seems unlikely that such recognition could be won by nursing in its present form, although it might fit more closely the definition of a 'semi-profession' like social work or teaching. Enormous energy is devoted to the definitions of a profession, usually developed by sociologists, and arguing about whether nursing fulfils the classic criteria (eg., practice being based on a recognised body of knowledge, control of entry, and conformity to a moral and disciplinary code). Such discussion may be academically interesting, but why is it so popular in nursing books and articles? Even if it could be proved that nursing did fulfil the criteria, nothing would change. We would still be as badly paid, and as powerless, and patient care would not change. The question we should ask is not 'Is nursing a profession?' but 'Should we want nursing to be a profession, and if so, what do *we* mean by it? What are we hoping to achieve, and is this the best way to go about it?'

Some commentators who say nursing will never be a profession, because its numbers are too great and its academic requirements too low, make a distinction between a profession and professionalism. Although nursing cannot be a profession in the traditional sense, it can aspire to 'professionalism', meaning better standards of practice achieved through improving training, raising entry requirements and changing attitudes. The process or strategy adopted to achieve the goals of professionalism is sometimes described as professionalisation.

The terms are not just hair-splitting. They do help to demonstrate that professionalisation is a distinct strategy, a chosen way of achieving certain goals. It is not the only or necessarily the best direction in which nursing could move. It is a move to try to win all sorts of goals ranging from better care to better pay, which may be linked in some ways but are not necessarily the direct and inevitable result of using such a strategy. There are other means of fighting for these ends which do not require the pursuit of professional status.

The uncritical adoption of 'professionalism' as a goal and a slogan is reinforced in the wards and schools in many ways. Students are led to believe that all good nurses believe in professionalism, and by inference that people and bodies such as trade unions who do not use the same strategy are greedy and self-seeking. This strengthens the hand of 'professional' organisations and undermines those who choose another approach; in other words, the notion of professionalism is used in a political way because it enhances the views and aims of one group at the expense of others — though many people do it without conscious intent.

In particular the words are used to justify or condemn certain kinds of behaviour which may have nothing to do with the quality of patient care or with other supposedly professional concerns. Condemning a particular incident or action by a student as 'unprofessional' labels her as a failure and as someone who is unworthy to be a nurse; it puts her outside the nursing community. Sometimes this happens in the clinical work context, but it is very often used in relation to behaviour outside work or in the broader arena of disputes about work conditions and similar incidents — the student who 'makes trouble' by arguing about an unpleasant off-duty rota or about missing meal breaks may be stamped as 'unprofessional' regardless of the quality of her work with patients.

One nursing student was told by a tutor that she was unprofessional because she was eating an apple while waiting to go into a lecture in the school of nursing. The tutor could have made it clear if there was a rule about not eating in the school, which at least offers the students the possibility of challenging the rule if they think it is petty and pointless, but to label the act as unprofessional is absurd. As it happened the nurse was an extremely competent, compassionate, if you like 'professional' worker — but even if she were not, the fact of her eating an apple in the school would be quite beside the point.

This is just one small example of the way the words are used every day — to confirm not just acceptance of a particular approach to nursing's future but to instil in new recruits the acceptance of the establishment's moral and behavioural code. It is important because it shows how the idea of professionalism includes a whole way of seeing, or ideology, which implies a lot more than is usually directly expressed. That student nurse was made to feel that her whole identity and competence as a nurse was called into question; 'professionalism' was used as a stick to punish her with. Similarly, nurses who go on demonstrations or express overt political views (of a left-wing rather than right-wing nature) are also said to be unprofessional, as the journals' correspondence columns show whenever there is industrial action in the NHS. This is a slovenly and cowardly way of expressing disagreement and it debases the positive implications of being professional — to the extent that some nurses feel the term is now unusable in any positive sense.

The professionalising strategy has been taken up not only by representative organisations like the RCN but by statutory bodies and other influential nurses, so it must be taken seriously. The reasons why it should have taken such a hold are interesting and complex, and we have only just begun to look at them critically instead of accepting the strategy as the natural and obvious way to proceed. The supporters of the professionalising strategy hold influential positions in the hierarchy, statutory bodies and professional organisations, giving them plenty of opportunity to publicise their views, but the negative implications are rarely discussed. On the basis that most nurses are familiar with the advantages claimed for becoming a profession, some of the less often aired opposing views are summarised here.

What's wrong with professionalism?

It's divisive

Most basic nursing care in and outside hospitals is given by untrained people, and probably always will be. The strategy pays little attention to the needs of those carers and even of those cared for; it is not good enough to assume that improving the status of trained nurses will automatically improve patient care, though it might. The professionalists identify with other groups such as doctors and physiotherapists rather than ancillary and auxiliary staff, relatives and patients.

While claiming to improve care, professionalism can instead strengthen the barriers between nurses and patients which damage relationships and inhibit the effectiveness of nursing care. The belief that access to the knowledge base of nursing should be strictly controlled may help to protect the public but it may also exclude them from acquiring that knowledge. Nurses get distinctly uneasy with a relative who wants to give her husband a blanket bath or a patient who wants to take his own drugs, as though their patch is being encroached on; there is no trust in other people's good intentions or common sense or caring skills.

This bid for exclusive control over nursing knowledge and skills extends to the treatment of auxiliaries. Much could be done to prepare them better for their work, but this would weaken the qualified nurses' claim to professional status — for if nursing auxiliaries were seen to be too good at their job, it would undermine the professionalists' arguments that they deserve more because they have a monopoly of skills.

The political demands of professionalism — for better pay, more status and so on — are inseparable from its effects on nursing work. The attempt to win recognition and its attendant material benefits for a selected group inevitably

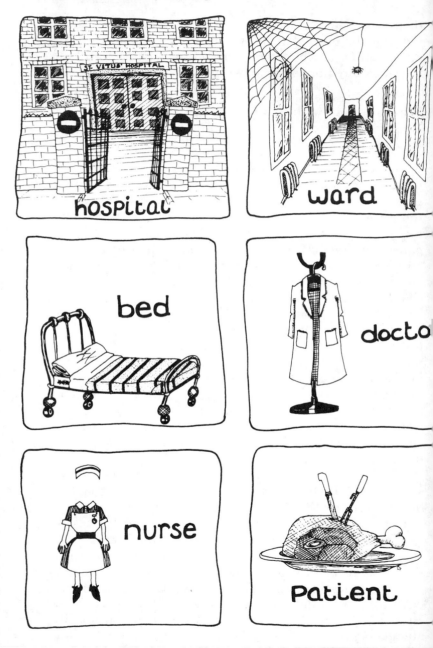

excludes others, and insisting on strict control of entry and education, and therefore knowledge, denies it to others, not least the patients themselves. The rarer your commodity, the more it is worth — ask Harley Street — but do we really want nursing to travel this road?

The elitism of the professionalism strategy in nursing has interesting roots in social class. Most nurses are from skilled working-class and lower middle-class backgrounds, and the desire to be upwardly mobile encourages them to draw a sharp distinction between themselves and working class employees like porters and auxiliaries (whose work is 'just a job'), while trying to ally themselves with successful middle-class workers like doctors. Bodies like the RCN love to adopt the gentility, formality and rituals which they perceive as characteristic of the upper middle classes, and this identification of middle-class values with professionalism leads to some heavy value-judgements. The RCN and its ilk are labelled as professional, patient-orientated, caring and good, while the TUC unions are supposed to be unprofessional, worker-orientated, selfish and bad.

Professionalism seeks to impose a uniform view of nurses

Professionalists tend to talk about 'the nursing profession' in the same way that the RCN calls itself 'the voice of nursing', implying a unified group of people who share the same aims. Nurses, they say, will be more powerful if they speak with one voice. Of course all nurses have some things in common, but there are also huge differences, as trade unionists/members of professional bodies, men/women, psychiatric/general nurses, managers/students, parents/childless people, and so on. In striving to establish a recognisable group identity, there is a danger of submerging real and important differences. The assumption that, say, managers and students should have the same goal — good nursing care — glosses over the fact that their positions are very different and that one is open to exploitation by the other. Nursing policies should be flexible, adaptable and realistic, not monolithic.

Professionalism denies the needs of its workers

Professionalism is not just an approach to nursing care, but implies an ethic which claims to put service to patients as its highest priority. It is largely concerned with improving the needs of a select group of nurses, while proclaiming an ideal of service before self — and it assumes those needs will be met by better status for the nurse, rather than by facing up to the problems most nurses face every day. Moreover, the emphasis on service is often used to discourage nurses from questioning the established order or taking matters into their own hands. The assertion that professionals do not strike is one example (though it is less often pointed out that they don't need to because they have high salaries); it is justified on the grounds that strikes harm patients, though the same voices have not been heard so forcefully on issues like the cuts, which harm far more patients than any strike. The dislike of industrial action has as much to do with fear of losing control and fear of being challenged as it does with caring about patients.

Professionalism emphasises an individual, not a collective approach

Recent assertions that nurses should individually be more accountable to patients and to other staff for their actions seem to be popular — the hierarchy's tendency to shift responsibility up or down has come under fire. The new ideas, though, put much emphasis on staff at ward level, where they seem to be expected to be accountable or responsible for situations in which they often have little control. The implications of encouraging them to be accountable primarily to patients rather than doctors have not been thought through, despite their enormous potential for conflict (in which the nurse is likely to come off worst). Accountability and the individualist approach of the nursing process may lay nurses open to blame and even disciplinary action, making it easier to find a scapegoat if things go wrong. This stress on individual responsibility, while in some ways welcome, also neglects the role and the possibility of acting together — suddenly, despite being part of 'the profession', you're on your own.

This denial of collective responsibility is clearly illustrated in the disciplinary procedures carried out by the statutory bodies. These are regarded as an important hallmark of professional status because they give a group of nurses the power to enforce certain standards of conduct among their colleagues. A typical example is cited in *Professional Discipline in Nursing* by Reg Pyne, who has had much involvement in the statutory bodies' disciplinary activities. He describes the case of an SRN who, under intolerable pressure from 'severe staff shortage' and working 'quite excessive hours to keep the unit going', was driven to taking sodium amytal — speed — to get through her work.

Her nurse managers, when they finally 'saw the full picture', were kind and helpful, Pyne reports. They channelled the nurse to 'appropriate medical help' and readily accepted that they had 'failed' her, although they felt obliged to report her to the GNC so 'her actions could be subject to consideration about her future as a registered nurse.' Yet if accountability were more than a stick with which to beat individual (more junior) nurses, surely those nurse managers should have been the ones sent before the GNC investigating committee. They had failed the nurse, and the patients; they had failed in their duty as managers to care for their staff and to ensure an adequate service was provided for patients. Through that failure the nurse suffered, and was made to suffer further from the trauma of a disciplinary case. Rather than sending her for 'medical help' to salve their consciences, they should have made immediate and forceful demands to the health authority for more staff — or closed the unit. It is their job to see the full picture.

Professionalism does not challenge the status quo

The changes in nursing care envisaged by the adherents of professionalism tend to support much of the status quo in health care. They tinker with what we already have, rather than taking a broader view and questioning whether the fragmentation of health care which is being accelerated by the developing autonomy of different professions is actually in the best interests of patients. It assumes that greater autonomy for nurses as a group will automatically benefit patients; it assumes that relatively few nurses should be highly trained and supervise larger numbers of untrained people; it does not even consider the idea of spreading education more widely to give a basic training to more people.

The professions fail to give strong support to the NHS

The vision of the future which professionalism presents to us is poor, mean and introverted. Instead of concentrating on vital questions like the future of the NHS and the need to protect what we have while trying to make improvements, it is more concerned with its own patch. Reading the documents of the RCN and the statutory bodies, you obtain remarkably little impression of serious thought about the health care system which underpins most paid nursing care. Indeed, professionalism may even draw nurses away from the NHS — for like the doctors, a professional nursing service could sell its skills more dearly in the market place (as a group of senior nurse managers, having learned their skills in the NHS, are already doing). This would dilute its commitment to improving the state-run health service and, as in medicine, would probably make it harder for patients to share in their care, to receive straight and full information or to make their own informed decisions.

Professionalism, then, is as much about pursuing the narrow interests of a particular group as it is about improving health care. In nursing it is an attempt to challenge medical power by aping medicine's methods, which in the long run may bring benefits to a few; highly qualified staff would be better paid and have more satisfying and prestigious jobs. But many questions need to be asked about its effects on others — unqualified staff, junior staff, other groups of workers, and patients.

So far there has been a marked failure within the nursing

establishment to explore or even discuss other possible approaches. It is true that issues such as accountability and the need for patient-centred care, often linked implicitly or explicitly to professionalism, do provide a chance to debate some of these vitally important assumptions about the job nurses do, about relationships with patients and about future patterns of health care — a debate to which I shall return later in this book. That debate is itself healthy, but it needs to be examined — its frame of reference widened and its terms used with greater precision. To offer a critique of professionalism in nursing is not to suggest that all those who pursue that ideal are greedy and self-seeking. But we should recognise that it is only one of a number of possible responses to the long-running health care crisis and the rapid changes in society and nursing itself.

Further Reading

Kennedy I. (1983). *The unmasking of medicine*. London: Paladin Books.

Oakley A. (1984). What Price Professionalism? The Importance of Being a Nurse. *Nursing Times*; December 12, pp. 24–7.

Pyne R. (1981). *Professional discipline in nursing*. Oxford: Blackwell.

Radical Nurses Group (1982). Nurses and nursing. A series of articles in *Medicine in Society*; **8 (4)**. Available from Central Books (Periodicals Dept.), 14 The Leathermarket, London SE1 3ER.

Williams K. (1974). Ideologies of nursing: their meanings and implications. *Nursing Times*, Occasional Paper; August 8.

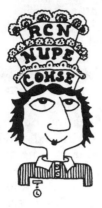

5

Getting organised

Professionalism, as we have already seen, has become a major preoccupation in nursing, and it is no coincidence that the name of the Royal College of Nursing — the major 'professional organisation' in the nursing arena — should crop up so often in that discussion. Whatever your views of professionalism, there is no doubt that the RCN has played a huge role in nursing's occupational development, and has contributed enormously to building a sense of pride in the job and to developing and safeguarding nurses' rights and welfare. It also works hard to spread knowledge and expertise, its associations and forums often providing the chief focus of interest and skills in specific areas of practice. It boasts an efficient legal and industrial relations service, and the combination it offers of professional enhancement and workplace protection is a strong recruitment incentive, reflected in its enormous claimed membership of a quarter of a million. Indeed, the college is the fastest growing union not affiliated to the TUC.

There is another side to the story, though, and one that is far less often heard. All nurses today can and most do belong to either a trade union or a professional organisation, or to both; and although nurses generally regard themselves as being apolitical or politically inactive, and regard some forms of political activity as unsuitable or unprofessional, trade unionism in nursing in fact has a long history — longer than that of the self-styled professional bodies. For instance, Mick Carpenter in *All for One*, part of his historical account of the Confederation of Health Service Employees, describes a strike by mental nurses over pay and conditions which took place in 1918, and other research is bringing to light similar examples of political action by nurses. So contrary to popular belief, or what some nurses and sections of the media would have us believe, the nurses who protested on picket lines in the 1982 NHS dispute were not a new phenomenon, but inheritors of a time-honoured tradition.

Widespread industrial action in the NHS is, however, relatively recent, and is attributable to the massive growth of the health service trades unions as well as to the continuing exploitation of low paid staff. Unlike many unions, those which represent NHS staff have managed on the whole to retain the large memberships they have attracted in the past 20 years or so. The increasing complexity, proliferating bureaucracy and long-distance management of the NHS have all encouraged the growth of the unions; managers no longer settle disputes on the spot but are likely to resort to formal procedures in which the unions have been more or less willing cooperators. Despite the media picture of callous, irresponsible and lazy strikers, large organisations like the NHS find the unions mostly useful partners in personnel management, a helpful means of contacting and controlling an unwieldy workforce.

Nurses have been no exception to this growth of trade unionism in the health service. COHSE, over half of whose members are nursing staff, fought for better nurses' pay by industrial action and demonstrations in 1950, 1962, 1970, 1973 and more recently. The National Union of Public Employees — a giant union with a third of its members in the NHS — has represented nurses since the 1930s and has been equally prominent in pay campaigns. Some nursing staff belong to other TUC unions like NALGO and GMBATU. Membership statistics are notoriously inaccurate, but even allowing for considerable inflation of their nursing members, it seems that getting on for half of the nursing staff in the

NHS (including qualified nurses, students and the untrained) belong to a TUC-affiliated union.

Nurses have always been willing to join trade unions, yet while those unions have always been concerned with protecting their members and improving their well-being through better pay and conditions, they have not been particularly concerned with the nature of nursing or with the issues now loosely called 'professional' ones, such as standards of care or education. Many nurses are therefore attracted to the professional organisations, which offer specialised educational services and a forum in which to debate such issues and present views to governments and policy-making bodies. Professional interests and personal welfare are not necessarily incompatible, but they have tended to be split between different organisations, often of diverse political colours. From their origins, the trade unions embraced socialist ideas — though not all were affiliated to the Labour Party — while the professional bodies were conservative and considered themselves a cut above the unions in terms of class and lack of self-interest; the broad differences hold good today, although the traditional distinctions are becoming increasingly blurred.

The history of the professional organisations, like that of the NHS unions, can be traced back to the early part of this century. By far the most powerful is the RCN, which claims to represent about 65% of all trained nurses and about 75% of nursing students, but excludes other (untrained) nursing staff from membership. Although it always had something to say about pay and conditions, the college's labour relations services were not extensively developed until the early 1970s, when it began to compete more vigorously with the unions for members in response to the growth in NHS unionisation. COHSE and NUPE were also introducing shop stewards and better local representation at this time, and the battle for members has continued unabated — fuelled by the knowledge that all the organisations desperately need members' subscriptions to fund their activities.

RCN membership has rocketed in the last 10 years, more than doubling since 1977. Like professional organisations in

'I'm studying nurses and their position in the labour force and the organisations they join. It's fascinating and complicated because they are at one and the same time workers and professionals and they come from such different class, racial and educational backgrounds; the auxiliary, the pupil nurse, the student, the ones doing nursing degrees, the 'mature' learners, the old-time nursing officers and the trendy sisters, the middle-aged enrolled nurses with families, the male nurses who have shot up the hierarchy, etc. etc.! A nurse's job is changing all the time — in relation to the doctor and other health workers and because of the increase in medical technology, the new ideas in nursing theory, the increased role of the state in terms of cuts in cash and policies about private medicine, and the whole role of medicine and the type of health care given in our society and the way it is beginning to be questioned . . .'

Nurse researcher

other occupational fields, it has come to recognise that professional and labour relations issues are often inseparable; standards of care, for instance, depend heavily on adequate staffing levels and this has long been a subject of management-union negotiation. Like many other white-collar organisations, it has sought and won certification as an independent trade union (in 1977) and has ballotted its members on the issue of affiliation to the TUC (turnout was low but a majority voted against the idea). Both moves are an indication of its recognition of the broader political arena and its desire to be more influential in trade union activities, both nationally and locally.

The fierce recruitment competition and the present Conservative government's restrictive anti-union legislation are encouraging closer alliances between the organisations. There has been talk of a merger between COHSE and NUPE to create one powerful union for all groups of NHS staff, while some of the smaller professional organisations are considering merging with larger ones, since it is difficult for them to provide the large range of services

The main organisations representing nursing staff

Note: The information is as accurate as possible but may be subject to change, especially membership numbers and subscriptions. For addresses, see Appendix.

Organisation	Eligible to join	Total claimed membership	Claimed nur membership
Association of Health and Residential Care Officers (AHRCO)	Nurses working in nursing homes	Very small	Very small
Association of Nurse Administrators (ANA)	Senior nurses	600	600
Association of Supervisors of Midwives	National Board-approved supervisors of midwives	250	250
Confederation of Health Service Employees (COHSE)	All NHS employees	230 709 (180 282 women 50 427 men)	130 000
Health Visitors Association (HVA)	Health visitors; community nurses (as associates)	15 400 (15 300 women 100 men)	15 400
Managerial Administrative Technical & Supervisory Association (MATSA)	White collar workers in all occupations	70 000	10 000
National & Local Government Officers' Association (NALGO)	White collar workers in all occupations	796 145 (408 820 women 387 325 men)	Small
National Union of Public Employees (NUPE)	Public sector employees	689 046 (459 364 women 229 682 men)	80 000
Royal College of Midwives (RCM)	Midwives	24 094	24 094
Royal College of Nursing (RCN)	Qualified nurses and those in training for a statutory qualification	240 000 (185 000 qualified 55 000 students)	240 000
Scottish Association of Nurse Administrators (SANA)	Senior nurses in Scotland	Very small	Very small
Scottish Health Visitors Association (SHVA)	Health visitors (including students) in Scotland	1000	1000

Main areas of nursing strength	Affiliated to the TUC?	Affiliated to the Labour Party?	Subscription
Nursing homes	Yes — through its link with NALGO	No	not available
Senior managers	No	No	£50/year
Midwifery	No	No	£5/year
Psychiatric and mental handicap nursing	Yes	Yes	£28.56/year
Health visiting	Yes	No	£42/year
General hospitals	Yes — it is the white collar section of the General, Municipal, Boilermakers & Allied TU	Yes	£38.40/year
Community, some managers	Yes	No	£37.44/year
Junior nursing grades	Yes	Yes	£26.04/year
Midwifery	No	No	£41.40/year
Most areas, especially general nursing; managers; students; teachers	No	No	qualified £45/year students £30/year
Managers in Scotland	No	No	£15/year
Health visitors in Scotland	No	No	qualified £45/year students £20/year

members demand. None of these plans is likely to reach fruition in the near future but they show how staff organisations of whatever constitution are constantly changing, adapting and seeking greater power, and the volatile nature of any assumptions we may make about their current state, status and political direction.

Why join anything?

Nurses join unions and professional bodies for a variety of reasons ranging from the desire to improve standards of care to dissatisfaction with their pay and working conditions. Some identify with the professional bodies' claim to be 'the voice of nursing' and their stated aim of putting patients first, while others are attracted by the unions' determination to fight for their members' interests. Local circumstances and traditions in particular places or types of work may also influence the nurse's choice, along with political sympathies and views on the ethics of industrial action. Whatever their motives, the vast majority of the 400 000 NHS nursing staff belong to something, but only a minority play an active part, suggesting that most join primarily for the protection offered by indemnity insurance or representation in disputes with senior staff.

In general the unions are assumed to have their members' interests as their first priority, while the professional bodies' main concern is supposed to be the development of the profession itself and the quality of care it provides, with the patient's interests coming first. This distinction is crude and inaccurate, although many people still seem to believe it and use it as a basis for their choice. In reality, the interests of the unions and professional organisations overlap considerably. Trade unions of all colours have done a great deal to improve workers' pay and conditions; nurses today rightfully complain that their wages are too low, but they would be considerably worse off without strong representative organisations. In the absence of that collective opposition, governments would get away with paying less and conditions would be far worse. History shows that improvements have come about not as a result of good will from people in high places, but through pressure from people united in unions — and prepared to use the availability of their labour as a bargaining counter.

People like nurses who work in the public sector are at a disadvantage here because they cannot claim a share of company profits; if they go on strike for more money, they do not harm their employers as much as they harm the people in their care — in fact, they save the government money. Although tactics of so-called 'industrial' action and union activity copied from worker organisations in factories and manual trades have increasingly been adopted in the NHS, on the whole staff have had to rely on the strength of their representation in the Whitley Councils, consisting of union and management representatives who negotiate how the money allotted to them by the government should be shared out. The 11 councils have also secured many improvements in working conditions, forcing NHS employers to conform to standards which they might otherwise have ignored, although government moves and dissatisfaction with the cumbersome machinery have recently led to a breakdown of Whitley — hastened by the establishment of the nurses' pay review body.

The hope of improving pay and conditions is a strong reason why nurses join unions. Membership also gives them an official way of expressing grievances and securing improvements locally; one nurse might feel powerless and too intimidated to protest about staff shortages on her ward to a senior nurse, but the union — presuming her stewards are active and effective — gives her an official, legitimate voice for her protest which also helps protect her from victimisation. More often, though, the unions are used negatively to defend members against mishap rather than positively to push for improvements.

This protective function of unions — defending its members when they are accused of misconduct — has a special dimension for nurses, whose work gives them unusually heavy responsibilities. One mistake with the simplest injection could cause permanent harm, and the growing tendency for patients and relatives to sue for damages after such incidents — combined with the desire of cost-conscious health authorities to off load the bill on to the individual practitioner — is making nurses feel more vulnerable and more aware of the need for protection.

The trend for nurses to assert themselves as independent practitioners, and the resulting claim that they are, therefore, directly accountable for their actions, has brought legal and insurance questions to the fore. Nurses working in the community, who are more likely to be practising independently, are showing a particular interest in indemnity insurance schemes to cover them against damages, and this is being looked at by organisations like the Community Psychiatric Nurses Association. Even bodies like COHSE which have traditionally argued that there was no need for such insurance are coming under growing pressure from nurse members, who feel they need more protection. NUPE quotes legal advice that although in theory a nurse could be personally sued for negligence, whether or not the employing authority was an additional defendant, this is most unlikely to happen in practice. Customarily action is taken only against the employer, and the employer or their insurers pay any damages. Other lawyers disagree and, unless more cases are contested in court and provide clear precedents, the area will probably remain grey.

The RCN and some other professional bodies meet the need for protection, or some would say exploit nurses' fears, by offering a comprehensive indemnity insurance scheme, which ensures that in most circumstances a member found guilty of professional negligence has her legal costs and any damages awarded against her underwritten by an insurance company. This increases the size of the subscription but many nurses choose to pay extra in return for the security they feel it offers. Many give the insurance scheme as their main reason for joining, and the RCN makes great play of it in its recruitment literature. Generally speaking, the TUC unions prefer to avoid such schemes and to sell themselves on their expertise in labour relations and the support they give members in trouble. All the organisations — professional and TUC — provide free legal advice to members and representation (of varying quality) at grievance hearings, tribunals, disciplinary committees and the like.

The unions are not just there for protection, though, and part of their attraction lies in their role as agents of social change. From the beginnings of the trade union movement, members recognised that their unity could give them a strong voice not only to improve their own standards of living, but to fight for benefits for the working class as a whole. The alliance between the union movement and the Labour Party helped to elect governments which created the modern welfare state, and in particular the NHS, giving health care to everyone regardless of class, status or union membership. Today those class allegiances and political links are less clear cut, but it remains true that the unions represent one of the strongest challenges to a government which is running down the NHS and encouraging private medicine.

Another longer term benefit of union/professional body participation is the opportunity that it gives for comment and consultation on broad social issues. Government policy documents on health care, for example, or the statutory bodies' plans to change nurse training, are sent to all the organisations for comment; there is no guarantee that their views will win the day but at least they can try, and the more members are involved, the greater the chance they will be able to affect the outcome. One of the reasons for the RCN's growing influence is its readiness to make its views known on nursing issues, and moreover to do the background work to make those views worth noting, an opportunity which the unions have so far failed to grasp fully as far as nursing is concerned.

Which one should I join?

The nurse who wants to join a trade union or professional organisation has a number of choices. Four TUC-affiliated unions have nurse members, and in addition to the RCN, the major professional body, there are specialist organisations which offer trade union-type benefits and professional services to particular groups, such as health visitors, managers, residential home nurses and midwives.

She may want to take a variety of factors into account. What are the aims and policies of the organisations? How well do they meet her needs — as a nurse in a particular field of work, as a part-timer, as a woman worker? What services are offered and how do the subscriptions compare? Will the organisation want her to take part in industrial action, and what are its political leanings?

One difficulty in choosing is that the advantages of each organisation depend to some extent on its strength in each place of work. You may decide that NUPE is the one for you, but there would be little point in joining it if everyone else belonged to, say, COHSE — unless they were all dissatisfied and felt that switching to the rival union was a good idea. Local strength of numbers is a major consideration, as an organisation with widespread local support is likely to have skilled stewards to represent the nurse and good links with full-time officials, and is more likely to carry weight with management. On the other hand, some union branches are dominated by autocratic local officials who may care little for the nurse's views — especially those officials who adopt the traditional view that nurses are apathetic and fail to support other health service workers. In those circumstances the nurse may feel deterred from joining — though changes will only happen if she is prepared to challenge such people and to put some effort into membership, seeing it as active rather than passive.

Some people feel that no one organisation representing nurses offers the range of services and commitment they need, and they solve the problem by holding joint membership. They may join the RCN for its professional services and nursing expertise, but also subscribe to COHSE or NUPE for their firmer commitment to the NHS, the contact with the other groups of staff and their labour relations skills. This means, of course, that they pay two subscriptions, which is a deterrent to people on low salaries.

One way of deciding which one the nurse wants to support

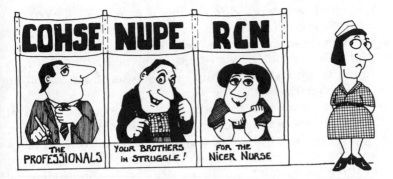

is to compare their record and attitudes on key points such as services offered, commitment to the NHS, industrial action and so on. Here we will look at the three which attract the most nurses and which compete directly for members — COHSE, NUPE and the RCN.

History

The origins of the three organisations tell us something about their current positions. The RCN was founded in 1916 on the initiative of a group of matrons and doctors, to follow the model of the Royal Colleges of Physicians and Surgeons and to press for the introduction of state registration of nurses. It received a Royal Charter in 1928, and still has royal patrons and a large list of titled non-nurses as vice-presidents. Although its aims are concerned with 'promoting the science and art of nursing' and 'the advance of nursing as a profession', it began to move away from its position as the voice of the matron élite (when it had supported positions such as keeping students' wages down) and to undertake more work in pursuit of the members' interests.

The college did not admit men till 1960 and is still trying to shake off the twin sets and pearls aura of ladylike respectability which now seems both outdated and unlikely to attract the monopoly nurse membership to which it aspires. COHSE, on the other hand, has its origins not in the teaching hospital matron élite but in the mental hospitals of the turn of the century, whose staff were not so much nurses as attendants and worked in very poor conditions for terrible wages. Through various name changes and mergers, it has retained its strong roots in mental nursing and was able to capitalise on the RCN's exclusion of men. It has always supported the NHS and from early on was affiliated both to the Labour Party and the TUC.

NUPE developed from the trade union organisation of municipal manual workers in the late 19th century, adopting its present name in 1928. Its membership has grown in leaps and bounds along with the public sector itself; recruitment of health workers dates back to the 1930s when county councils controlled some health services. In the 25 years when Alan Fisher was general secretary, up till 1982, its membership increased by half a million to just over 700 000, boosted by the local interest generated by the introduction of its shop steward scheme in 1968.

Eligibility

Much of the RCN's present strength derives from the fact that its membership is restricted to qualified nurses and those in training; nursing auxiliaries are excluded, by conference decision. This enables it to concentrate single-mindedly on nurses and nursing, and certainly the organisation has been very successful in representing views on nursing issues to civil servants and statutory bodies, showing an impressive and convincing knowledge of the field. Its claim to speak for 'the profession' has been used by governments when it suits them — such as in the 1982 dispute, when the Conservatives falsely claimed that nurses, unlike other health workers, were refusing to take industrial action and that the pay review body was a reward for a no-strike pledge. However, the RCN's failure to secure exclusion of auxiliaries from the remit of the pay review body shows that the government is prepared to ignore 'the profession', as expressed through the RCN, when it chooses.

The enormous strength of the college among qualified staff — including, probably, most senior managers and teachers as well as many sisters — can lead it to take a narrow view of health care. Although it is becoming more vociferous about the problems of the NHS, its statements fail to emphasise that health care is actually teamwork, and that standards do not depend on nurses alone. In representing its members' interests it feels no particular obligation to support NHS staff who are even worse paid than nurses, and indeed it insists on maintaining the gap between nurses and those below them as part of its strategy of professionalisation.

Both COHSE and NUPE, in contrast, draw their strength from the massive size and diversity of their memberships. The opportunity they offer for porters and nurses to rub shoulders with domestics and ambulance personnel does much to help each group understand the others' problems and preoccupations. COHSE has some advantages over NUPE in that all its members work in the health service, so it can concentrate on NHS affairs. In some ways it represents the best of both worlds, with a varied membership but a majority of nursing staff (about 55%) including many qualified nurses and some in managerial posts. Many of its full-time officials, including the general secretary, worked as nurses before moving into the union.

COHSE is the fastest growing union in the TUC but in recent years it has faced a strong challenge from the giant public sector union NUPE, which also has members in local authorities (such as refuse collectors and parks attendants), universities and water authorities, mostly in manual jobs. NUPE's militant stance, especially in disputes, has attracted many health service workers, although its base in manual labour has led many nurses to prefer COHSE, which seems to combine a commitment to trade unionism with a more informed interest in professional nursing issues. Nonetheless it is one of NUPE's strengths that it places its attitudes to the NHS and health care firmly in the broader social and political context. Of the three organisations, it is the only one which has comprehensive and positive policies to encourage the involvement of its female members (two thirds of the total); recently it appointed a former ward sister as national women's officer to help put these policies into practice.

NUPE's nursing members are only about 10% of the total and the proportion of qualified nurses is probably far smaller, so it is not surprising that the union fails to speak strongly on nursing issues, generally commenting only in very broad terms. Its nurse members also face what the union itself describes as 'traditional barriers' between them and other grades of staff; in many branches dominated by ancillary workers, there is a failure to understand why nurses find it more difficult to attend meetings in work time or to join wholeheartedly in strike action. Nevertheless it sees nursing as a fertile recruitment field and is developing better policies through its nurses' advisory committee.

Membership strengths

Traditionally COHSE is strong in psychiatric and mental handicap hospitals and much of the work it has done on nursing has concentrated on this area. Its obligation to

---

'We have a number of nurse members but most of them don't want to get active, either because they are apathetic or frightened of management or feel whatever they do has no effect. I have to battle away on the basis that if I don't things will be even worse! Gradually people become more interested if I keep them informed and organise meetings — I do this monthly and only nurses can come because I feel they have unique problems not applicable to ancillary staff because of the nature of their work. Nurses need to feel they are supported in this way. We discuss pay and conditions and individuals' problems, but I don't go for all this political stuff. I do encourage my members to go to general branch meetings too. Even if only a few people are active at first, it can have a snowball effect as it has in other psychiatric hospitals. Though I'm blowing my own trumpet, I am hard working and efficient and enthusiastic as a local steward, and this is the main factor in the quality of the union here.'

COHSE steward — psychiatric nurse

protect its members' interests has led to some sticky situations, with COHSE members and branch officials accused of closing ranks to cover up the abuse of patients by nurses. Government policies to shift resources away from long-stay hospitals to 'community care' have put the confederation in the awkward situation of having to defend an apparently reactionary attitude — in defence of the long-stay hospitals — because its RMN and RNMH members fear, probably with justification, that their jobs may simply disappear and that the much-promised resources for community care will never materialise.

The RCN has presented a challenge to COHSE by setting up a society of psychiatric nursing, serviced by a full-time official, to cater for the interests of mental nurses, and more recently a similar society for nurses in mental handicap. But the failure of both organisations to meet the needs of this neglected group is illustrated by the founding of the Psychiatric Nurses Association — not a trade union, but a response to mental nurses' desire for an autonomous organisation and also part of a general tendency towards fragmentation into specialist groups.

The college now offers an enormous range of societies, forums and associations to meet special needs, which have undoubtedly enhanced its attraction to nurses in every field.

'I joined NUPE because the RCN is not very interested in pay and conditions or the future of the NHS. It is not as militant as NUPE, but contrary to the popular image NUPE members are not callous and money-grabbing — if we don't fight for better pay, staffing levels will fall even further and patients will suffer — as they will if the NHS is taken over by the private sector. At my hospital NUPE has separate, regular meetings for nurses and is more active than the RCN — and it gives me more contact with ancillary workers and helps me to see their viewpoint. I realise my NUPE membership causes some hassles at work but I feel I can cope with it.'

Student nurse

There are alignments of, say, all nurses in the community and all nurses in occupational health, and other groupings of managers, clinical nurses, students and educationalists. All the groups have their own networks, publicity, conferences, study days and representation at the RCN's annual delegate conference, and all help to provide and spread the specialist knowledge which makes the college such a strong and reliable commentator on nursing issues.

NUPE's attraction for nurses is of a different kind. It offers nursing auxiliaries the advantages of forceful local representation and commitment to improving conditions for the low paid, but it also attracts students and trained nurses who have firm political leanings to socialism and so provide a good core of committed activists. Recently NUPE has tended to attract many graduate nurses, who like its pro-NHS views and feel alienated by the aspirant middle-class respectability of the RCN and the old-fashioned labourism and sexism of COHSE.

Politics

NUPE and COHSE are both affiliated to the TUC and the Labour Party, and sponsor Labour MPs (paying a proportion of their election expenses), which gives them direct access to Parliament. Part of each member's subscription is paid into Labour Party funds unless the individual specifically asks to be excluded from this 'political levy' (now likely to be abolished by the government). Officials of both unions hold senior Labour Party positions and their members on the TUC General Council give them an important voice within the labour movement, though they have had their differences with Labour health ministers.

In recent years the public sector unions have worked for more cooperation and a united front in response to wage restraints and anti-union laws. The 1982 NHS dispute showed unprecedented unity between the unions on the TUC health services committee, which coordinated industrial action throughout the country. This had the effect of undermining the most extreme action, since the more moderate unions held back the hard-liners, but it also helped to forge links between unionists at the grass roots, for example by the establishment of new joint shop stewards' committees.

This TUC committee also plays a less publicised role in helping to develop the TUC's policies on health care. The influence of the TUC is still strong and is acknowledged by many white-collar unions who now wish to join (in the past they have regarded it with antipathy). A minority in the RCN have pushed for TUC affiliation but have been unsuccessful, partly because of misconceptions about the TUC's powers (some nurses think TUC membership means they will be forced to strike). They have, though, been heartened by the entry of other 'professional organisations' and some people argue it is only a matter of time before the college applies for affiliation — a move which would be strongly opposed by NUPE and COHSE, since it would increase their rival's influence.

The TUC is also a useful source of educational and political activity and material. It runs courses on negotiation, health and safety, women's rights, employment law, using the media and so on which are open to affiliated unionists and give them a chance to mix and compare notes with members from different work situations. Many of its publications are attractive and informative, such as its workbook on the Black report, *Inequalities in Health*.

The RCN, in contrast to COHSE and NUPE, claims to have no political allegiances. Its label as a moderate, politically centrist organisation is based on its general ethos as well as on specific policies; its refusal to oppose private medicine, or recent legislation on unions, and its belated entry into the campaign against cutbacks, reflects such leanings. Politics have long been meat and drink to most COHSE and NUPE activists but RCN members are only just beginning to learn that a concern for standards of nursing care will inevitably draw them into political discussion and action, though not necessarily of a party political type. The growing, if ill understood, feeling that nurses need 'political awareness' is reflected in the college's recent appointment of a parliamentary liaison officer.

Democracy

Trade union democracy is a lively issue. None of these three organisations can claim to be more democratic than the others (although they all do), though they have differences; as in other groups the minority of active members have a large say in policy, and the full-time officials dominate. All three have annual conferences where resolutions from the branches are discussed and voted on, forming the basis of the union's policy; in theory COHSE and NUPE's conferences, with delegates from all branches, are the supreme governing bodies, while in the RCN that authority is vested in a council elected every four years. In practice, though, the leadership of the organisations — an alliance between full-timers and some prominent members — can and sometimes does overrule conference decisions, or modifies them in the light of events.

COHSE distinguishes itself by electing its general and deputy general secretaries from among its members, though this takes place through the branches rather than individual postal ballot; in the other two the general secretary is appointed by the members' council. Consultation in NUPE and COHSE tends to take place through the branches, which may put members at a disadvantage if they cannot get to meetings or if the branch secretary is inactive. The RCN branches, called centres, are generally less active and often concentrate on educational or social activities; consultation on vital issues increasingly takes the form of individual postal voting, which gives a more accurate picture of the membership's views. In 1982 RCN members twice voted in this way to reject the government's pay offer (to the surprise of many).

The RCN has often been accused of being dominated by managers. This may be less true nowadays, though its council still has a disproportionate lack of clinical practitioners, and many senior nurses sit on its committees and boards. As the organisation has grown in numbers and confidence, there is increasing pressure on it to pay more attention to the problems and concerns of the ordinary working nurse. The presence of nurses of all grades in local meetings often inhibits free discussion, however, as junior and student nurses are inevitably less vociferous in the company of other members who may be their seniors in education or service. NUPE and COHSE nurses face problems of a different kind in that the nursing viewpoint may go unheard in branches where ancillary staff dominate.

Attitudes to industrial action

No union, including those in the TUC, can force its members to do anything, and in the NHS even the chances of being expelled from a branch for refusing to take industrial action are remote. COHSE and NUPE nurses have taken such action and will continue to do so, but both unions recognise the special position of people involved in direct patient care and have enshrined it in codes of practice; apart from occasional circumstances where labour relations have broken down completely or where the members are very militant, withdrawal of labour is never complete, with 'emergency cover' being provided to protect patients.

In practice, of course, life is not so simple. The row about whether nurses can and should withdraw their labour under any circumstances has been gathering steam, and reached a climax with the notorious General Nursing Council statement of 1979. Supposedly intended to clarify the nurse's position on industrial action, in fact it intensified the disagreement although it did at least succeed in putting the issue on the official agenda. The statement, condemned by COHSE and NUPE in the strongest possible terms, said that a nurse who participated in industrial action might have 'a case to answer on the score of professional misconduct' if the action put the health, safety or welfare of patients at risk.

All the statement did on the face of it was reiterate the GNC's legal obligation to protect the public by demanding certain standards of conduct of the qualified nurse. But even if the council's motives were honourable, there is no doubt that some nurse managers used it as a threat to deter possible action: 'If you go on strike, the GNC will strike you off.' There would in fact be no question of this automatic removal from the register or roll, as each case is heard individually and judged on the particular circumstances.

The increasing willingness of nurses to participate in industrial action — not only over pay rises, but on issues such as staff cuts and hospital closures — has made the question of industrial action perhaps the most bitter division of all in nursing today. Inside the RCN, which has a traditional no-strike policy, attempts have been made (unsuccessfully) to abolish Rule 12, which effectively rules out strikes and lays down particular conditions under which industrial action could be called by its council. Some nurses argue that unless they take such action they will remain powerless, while others argue that the moral commitment not to strike is nurses' strongest weapon. Events have not proved either side to be right; the no-strike pledge has not yet been rewarded financially by any government, despite the claims made for the pay review body, while industrial action has failed to secure significant gains — though its supporters say this is because it has never been used on a wide enough scale.

NUPE's nurses advisory committee has provided examples of the protest action nurses could take 'which whilst being effective, would safeguard the welfare of patients in the direct care situation'. These suggestions, which are very similar to those drawn up by an RCN action committee but never implemented, include:

- refusal to admit patients other than emergencies.
- the banning of all overtime work.
- strict application of clinical nursing duties.
- strict application of shifts.
- refusal to act up or down.
- insistence on all wards being staffed by trained nurses at all times.

Some nurses argue that such action could be taken not only over their own pay, but to protest at staff shortages. They say industrial action in such circumstances should be seen as a professional responsibility in the patient's interests, ultimately; otherwise nurses will continue 'coping' with too few resources and standards will continue to fall.

Services offered

All the organisations have full-time officials in each health region, to keep the branches in touch and provide expert support for the lay officials (those who work in the NHS). Generalisations are difficult because so much depends on the individual. The RCN undoubtedly has the edge in servicing its members on clinical matters; each area has a full-time 'nurse adviser' concerned specifically with professional rather than labour relations matters, and each adviser also services one of the specialist societies (primary care, psychiatry, cancer nursing and so on).

This mix of functions which is one of the college's great attractions is also displayed in its weekly newspaper *Nursing Standard*, free to members, which carries articles on nursing policy, current issues and professional matters. COHSE and NUPE have regular journals which carry far less material of specific nursing interest. RCN members also meet each other at study days, courses, conferences and seminars, which play an important role in creating a sense of belonging to an organisation which cares about nursing practice — an advantage the others lack.

What's wrong with them all

Traditionally trade unions are seen as organisations dominated by working-class men — the old cloth-cap image. This is not only out of date, but is particularly inappropriate for the NHS, most of whose staff are women. NUPE and COHSE have a majority of women members, yet most of their top posts are occupied by men and many branch officials are men: the people in charge may have little understanding of the needs and problems of their women members. Many women working in the NHS are also responsible for looking after children, so they may be unable to go to evening meetings or take on the onerous duties of being an official or an activist. The unions are quite happy to recruit them, but make relatively little effort to meet their needs by timing meetings differently, or organising creches or babysitters, or even by discussing the issue and its implications at local level. Union meetings can in any case be depressing and difficult for a woman. She may have to cope with sexist, patronising comments if she tries to speak, and she may find the traditional masculine way of conducting meetings, with rules (bent to the chairman's pleasure), order books and confusing jargon making her feel an outsider rather than one of the group. Many more women are now becoming active and have helped overcome these problems by getting together to support each other, such as by running women-only courses. Black women face even greater problems of acceptance by the traditional male trade unionist.

Both unions, mindful that most of their members are women and that women will be their main source of recruitment, and pressurised by vociferous female members, have started to encourage more female participation. NUPE (42% of shop stewards are women; two-thirds of members; six female area officers out of 127; five reserved seats on 26-strong executive committee) has appointed a national women's officer, and its women's working party — set up to identify the obstacles which prevent women from becoming more active — is working on issues like abortion rights and sexual harassment which are only just beginning to be taken seriously by the union movement.

COHSE (75% female membership; one female national officer out of six; a sprinkling of female full-time officials) has a less impressive record than NUPE on women's issues. So far there are few signs of change despite the efforts of some members to modify its macho pose — illustrated in a recent national conference row, when some officials and delegates ignored or ridiculed women members' protests about a 'Miss COHSE' beauty contest. Its membership contains fewer of the young left-wing militants who tend to be in the forefront of pressure for change on issues like sexism and racism, and who have helped to get things moving in NUPE.

The RCN likewise has paid remarkably little attention to the needs of its female members, perhaps surprisingly in an organisation which until recently was run almost exclusively by women and which has always had a huge majority of women in membership. Its old matron elite, mostly unmarried and middle class, had little sympathy with or awareness of the problems faced by poorly paid nurses trying to raise children and failed to throw its weight behind measures specifically aimed at helping women. Now that elite is being replaced by ambitious male managers and teachers who on the whole are equally unconcerned about the daily reality of the members' lives. The impact of feminism has forced it to modify its tune and has brought a greater awareness of these issues, but there is a long way to go. Its pay campaigns, for instance, have rarely highlighted the link between nurses' low pay and the low pay of women in general.

Criticisms of these bodies are often met with a comment about the leaders only carrying out the instructions of the members, and policies simply reflecting the general membership viewpoint. It is argued that the democratic channels exist in every organisation for those seeking change; while this is true in one sense it brushes aside the real obstacles to activity which most women face in their daily lives — how many men are prepared to look after the children while their spouse attends a weekend executive meeting in another city? The hierarchical structure of nursing presents another kind of obstacle, the domination of junior by senior nurses even outside the work relationship, leading to a reluctance by juniors to put themselves forward or express 'controversial' views. And while the union leaders should of course be the mouthpiece of the members' views, they also have a responsibility to initiate change, and have often been found sadly lacking in particular spheres, especially their concern for women.

The gap between the realities of the working life and the policies and activities of union/professional body leaders is not only a product of the different circumstances of the leaders and the led, though. It is part of the overall process of British political life, which gives the ordinary person little say in matters of vital importance. It reflects a situation in which the leaders address governments on complex and high-powered policy matters while workers worry about overtime pay or the shortage of clean uniforms. After a hard day's work, most people are understandably unwilling to give their precious free time to attending meetings or writing documents. Above all the gulf may reflect the power structure of a society where decisions are made far away by someone else, not by the people most affected.

This chapter started by observing that most nurses do in fact belong to either a union or a professional organisation, a situation which shows no sign of ending. In particular, the TUC unions' importance in health care is reaching a plateau, while the RCN strides on ahead. Yet the reasons have barely been discussed, since all sides usually have an axe to grind. This membership trend is one we can see in society as a whole, involving the upward social mobility of lower middle-class white-collar workers, and their subsequent desire to distance themselves from the working class — now backed by a government which is only too keen to foster the division and break one of the biggest threats to its power. The health unions have not been immune from the crisis facing the trade union movement as a whole, despite the NHS membership boom. Their power is weakened during a time of high unemployment, further eroded by anti-union laws and the hostile media, and in a shifting political climate they can no longer command such a strong base of traditional support.

In the present climate it is hardly surprising that organisations like the RCN, which are not aligned with the labour movement and which offer services involved with the professional aspirations of a particular class, should fare better. With the confidence gained through strength, it is voicing increasingly critical views of the government, which is perhaps not finding the college as firm an ally as it might once have expected. Hitherto the RCN has shown a depressing reluctance seriously to tackle major health issues such as NHS funding, but now — perhaps because senior nurses feel they themselves are under threat through new management policies — it is finding a stronger voice.

The picture is a confusing one for the nurse trying to work out where her sympathies lie. All the organisations have something to offer, but all have drawbacks too. Membership of anything is a sensible move in the face of possible redundancies, litigation, changing job descriptions and the erosion of rights at work, just as the collective strength of these organisations is an important brake on governmental excesses. Ultimately the strength of the organisation at local level may be the most important factor in situations where the nurse's job, pay or conditions are on the line, and at local level that strength depends on the members. Nurses who are prepared to join with others and take positive action on issues they think matter are more likely to succeed than those who remain isolated and alone.

Radical alternatives

Alongside the shifting loyalties of nurses between unions and professional bodies, another trend is becoming apparent — the proliferation of radical and specialist groups. They are diverse in nature and have varied origins, but all share a dissatisfaction with the ability of the existing bodies to meet their needs, and they also indicate the growing confidence of nurses in being prepared to act on their own initiative.

The groups fall broadly speaking into two categories — one concerned with developing the nurse's specialist clinical expertise, and the other concerned more with politics. Some, like the Association of Radical Midwives and the Psychiatric Nurses Association, combine both areas of interest and are probably all the stronger as a result. Some challenge the establishment not only in the topics they discuss, but in the way the group is organised, although none claims to offer an alternative to the established bodies. Some nurses (especially those allied to the RCN) lament this 'fragmentation' and claim that it dilutes and weakens the nursing voice, but others see it as a healthy sign of independence.

Some of the newer groups have sprung up around particular clinical interests. Nursing has followed medicine in becoming increasingly specialised, and like doctors, nurses working in a specific field are finding a need to meet and exchange information and views; newsletters, conferences and committees soon follow. The RCN, always looking for new members and ways of attracting them, regards itself as the natural home of such groups and the last two or three years have seen the launch of many new societies and forums within the college — some have grown from members getting together with a common interest in family planning nursing or stoma care, while others have been set up in response to a challenge from outside. Starting a group with no resources is a struggle and the college can offer funds and facilities, though the link is not always trouble-free. Interestingly, COHSE too is now pursuing this line in an attempt to boost membership and improve its services, and is hoping to establish special interest groups — a move which would have been howled down as divisive some years ago, but which is now seen as a sensible adaptation to changing circumstances.

A challenge to the traditional domination by general nurses of the nursing establishment, in both professional and statutory bodies, is implicit in some of the new groups. Midwives and health visitors, with different historical traditions and a discrete area of professional practice, have been able to preserve their separate organisations, though with some difficulty, and the price they paid has been a defensive conservatism. The issue is less clear cut for psychiatric and mental handicap nurses, but recent fears that their training may be reduced simply to a module in general training, with the full basic psychiatric training disappearing, have impelled them to start new groups or strengthen the older ones dealing specifically with their interests. The establishment of the new statutory bodies and the elections to the national boards provided an opportunity to raise such issues in public campaigning, and members of both the Radical Midwives and the Psychiatric Nurses Association were elected — indeed radical midwives swept the board in the English elections.

The new clinically oriented groups, and those dominated by men, tend to be organised in traditional ways, but the other 'radical' groups pose a challenge to tradition not just in the subject matter of their meetings but in the way the groups are organised and the meetings conducted. The Radical Midwives, Radical Nurses and Radical Health Visitors groups all organise themselves on a non-hierarchical, informal basis in a conscious attempt to bypass the traditional nursing structure and to promote a truly egalitarian atmosphere, in which even the most shy and nervous members feel able to speak their thoughts and feelings. They work through nationwide networks of members, often communicating through friendship and personal contact rather than more formal channels, and power and decision-making are vested firmly at the membership level, not centralised in remote committees. As far as possible the organising tasks — producing newsletters, running meetings, organising conferences and so on — are shared among all the members, to develop people's confidence and ability to do these things and to demystify the skills involved; shared responsibility also tends to mean shared power.

The impetus behind these groups is a sense of disillusionment with the job and frustration at the lack of opportunity to talk about problems openly — a pervading sense that nurses are not being listened to, either by peers and seniors at work or by the existing nursing organisations. 'As nurses we are not encouraged to examine our work or to share our doubts and frustrations,' say the Radical Nurses. 'Instead our training actively discourages us from discussing our work critically and makes us see the problems as individual

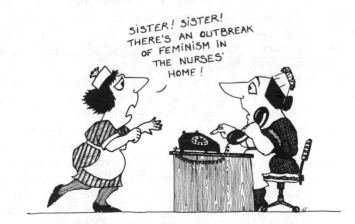

failings rather than as the responsibility of all nurses, of the NHS and of society as a whole.' The Radical Midwives decided 'to meet regularly to offer support and encouragement', with the greatest value to each other being 'study and support'.

While the groups are very critical of the established organisations, they see themselves more as ginger groups than as rivals. Their links and loyalties lie as much, if not more, with people who use health services as with 'the professions' and most members have great doubts about the direction in which 'professionalism' is going. The consensus is that belonging to a union is valuable and important, but members also want major changes in the bodies' concerns and in the way they are organised — often along the lines of the criticisms I have offered in this book, although there is no 'party line' or unanimous view on any topic, and debate and dissent is actively encouraged.

The agenda of the meetings shows a different range of interests and concerns from the usual content of an RCN or RCM meeting, or a trade union branch. Nursing as 'women's work', racism, the social causes of ill health, the health implications of nuclear war and the needs of the nurse as an individual are typical topics and the discussion is firmly rooted in personal experience as well as more theoretical points. Discussing and writing about such topics not just in meetings but also in hospitals and health centres up and down the country has helped to put them on the establishment agenda and to promote the recognition that they are legitimate concerns for nurses, although many people still see them as somewhat subversive!

One of the interesting things about the radical groups is the emergence of a core of articulate, well-educated nurses, midwives and health visitors with similar views as a new influence in the professions. A high proportion of them are graduates and/or people who have come to nursing later in life, with their ideas already formed; they are far less susceptible to the conditioning and far more likely to have the confidence to challenge the system or question dubious practices — which does not endear them to many others.

Through dissatisfaction a number have left nursing to work in allied health or social service jobs, while others are doing research into nursing, often from a sociological perspective. Unlike many of the old guard, they have friendships outside nursing which broaden their outlook and bring some fresh air into the stuffy corridors. Their views are increasingly publicised in the nursing press and at conferences, and some are moving into positions of responsibility which give them greater influence.

More than the other two groups, the Association of Radical Midwives has succeeded in attracting members who are probably more typical of the 'average' midwife (if there is such a creature). Conference attendance equals that of the major organisations and there is a network of over 20 regional contacts, with a large active membership. To some extent this is attributable to the more specific aims of the group and the general resurgence of interest, from lay people as well, in childbirth and the midwife's role; altogether it is a healthy growth and a vigorous and fruitful example for the other newer groups, showing that it is possible to discuss 'radical' ideas without frightening people away.

It is impossible to assess how far the radical groups are a consequence or a cause of some of the subtle changes taking place in nursing today — changes for the better — but they are undoubtedly playing a part, not least in reminding the traditional organisations, whether trade unions, professional associations or statutory bodies, of other concerns and other ways of working. They emphasise that the welfare of each nurse and patient is not just a personal matter but is part of a continuum or mesh of forces ranging from professional power politics through to economic policies and the status of women.

Pay: a case study in nursing politics

Nurses' pay — or the lack of it — is the one issue which unites everyone. Almost every nurse, except those in the top posts, would agree that present salaries are inadequate, not only in relation to what other workers receive but as recompense for the demands of a tiring and difficult job, in which they are expected to give of themselves mentally and physically and, often, to provide a round-the-clock service — regardless of the effects on their personal lives.

Added to this is the knowledge that most nurses can never expect to improve their earnings substantially despite gaining more experience, spending more years in the job or acquiring more qualifications. The ward sister, for example, is the pivot of the ward team for all disciplines involved in patient care; she will have had at least five years' experience of nursing and may hold additional qualifications or demonstrate specialist knowledge from courses and diplomas; yet her pay scale starts at only £6827. Running a car or paying a mortgage is a luxury, not the basic necessity expected in the wage levels of other jobs demanding similar levels of training and expertise. Even with increments she can earn a maximum of only £8751 until the day she retires from that post.

The picture is similar in education and management, where nurses on the whole are paid less than people doing comparable jobs in other fields. This is in itself unjust, but it also has the effect of driving people out of the occupation — the knowledge that any amount of hard work and development of expertise will not be financially recognised is a great disincentive, and is reflected (for example) in the recruitment problems besetting nursing education. Why become a nurse teacher when you may actually have to take a drop in salary from your previous post as a sister? Nurse managers receive little sympathy from the rest of the profession but they too have legitimate financial grievances, especially in the lower grades. For years district nursing officers were paid less than managers in other NHS disciplines such as doctors and finance officers, despite being described as equals in consensus management teams, and even now they receive less than others doing comparable jobs outside the public sector.

There is a feeling that nurses' pay is low in absolute terms, born of the experience shared by all nurses of making ends meet on a low budget, doing agency work to pay for holidays abroad or suffering the humiliation of being unable to afford clothes or entertainment enjoyed by friends in other jobs. It is common, however, to turn to the idea of comparisons in the search for hard evidence. The question of comparability had been central to pay campaigns in the last ten years — comparing yourself to another group of better paid workers is an obvious way of trying to persuade governments that your own group is disadvantaged. There is hard evidence that nurses' pay has failed to keep pace with that of other groups despite the occasional large rises which follow bursts of protest activity. At Aberdeen University researchers concluded that movement in nurses' pay over the last 30 years follows a clear pattern — a period of relative decline followed by a 'catching-up' award. Over 30 years the pay in real terms of trained nurses in fact rose by only 9%.

Comparing nursing with other jobs, though, does not automatically produce the desired results; it may strengthen the case but of itself it does not dazzle governments into giving huge increases. In any case using comparisons can be a two-edged weapon, since the choice of comparators is a matter of opinion. Nursing is a difficult job to quantify, as it contains so many different tasks and can vary so much from one specialty to another, and the occasional attempt to produce a list of comparators, or jobs it can be compared with, is always greeted with outrage. In 1982, for example, NHS management negotiators drew up a list of comparisons which included air hostesses and post office engineers, and in 1977 the DHSS attempted to break down the components of nursing jobs in the *Job Evaluation* report — both efforts proving highly unpopular.

Nonetheless, comparability has been and will probably continue to be a factor in pay negotiation. Sometimes it has been used as a successful basis for securing better deals — the Clegg commission which based its recommendations for pay increases on comparisons persuaded the government to award rises, though of course not as much as everyone would have liked. In some areas it produced comparisons which were held to be acceptable, such as that between ward sisters and house officers, adopting the sensible approach that

Nurses' pay — the history

- *The Halsbury Report, 1974*

  This was commissioned by Barbara Castle, then Labour social services secretary, following persistent action by nurses over pay, ranging from industrial action by COHSE and NUPE to the RCN's propaganda campaign 'Raise the Roof'. Halsbury's committee concluded that 'the pay of nurses and midwives has fallen below other occupations and professions which, four years ago, were at broadly similar levels'. Its recommendations were accepted by the government, and fully funded, giving nurses an average rise of 30%. But nurses again began to slip down the pay league — partly through the operation of incomes policies and partly through inability or reluctance to put on pressure through industrial action.

- *The Speakman Report, 1979*

  Top nurses rarely had much sympathy from the rest in their claims, although their wages compared unfavourably with other NHS disciplines on the 'teams of equals' at health authority level. The Speakman report, however, awarded substantial rises to regional, area and district nursing officers, based on parity with other managers.

  Nurses in general settled for 9% in that year's pay round (the going rate for the public sector), and a referral of their claim to Professor Hugh Clegg's Standing Commission on pay comparability set up by the Labour government.

- *The Clegg Commission, 1980*

  To complete the 1979 award, Clegg's third report recommended an extra rise averaging 19·6%. This ranged from 25% for sisters to nothing for top posts. The annual settlement was held to the NHS cash limit of 14% — all nurses received 13%, with the extra 1% shared among senior nurses. And for 1980–1 the government set aside £116 million to fund the shorter 37½-hour working week, representing 6% of the total wages bill.

- *The 1982 dispute*

  In 1981 the staff side accepted a 6% rise in line with cash limits, though it claimed 15% to keep up with inflation. The following year the government announced a ceiling of 4% for everyone except doctors, and the staff side claimed 12% in line with inflation. The enormous resistance to the low offer, with growing militancy among nurses and unprecedented unity between the unions, provoked the longest lasting and most widespread dispute ever seen in the NHS. This only came to an end in December, when nurses eventually and reluctantly accepted a 12·3% rise over two years, coupled with the promise of a new pay review body.

- *The Pay Review Body*

  After further delay and a brief period of consultation with nursing organisations, the government announced the composition and remit of the pay review body in July 1983. It determines the pay not only of nurses and midwives but also of other professions allied to medicine, such as physiotherapists and radiographers. Chaired by Sir John Greenborough, a former chairman of the Confederation of British Industries, it has a panel of independent members who assess evidence presented by interested parties — including the government, which will submit evidence on 'economic and financial considerations and such factors as recruitment, retention and motivation of staff'. The body will then recommend pay rises (which the government is not bound to implement).

job-for-job comparison was not necessarily appropriate but that elements of jobs could be separated out and subjected to analysis and comparison for pay purposes (known as 'factor analysis').

Why is nurses' pay so low?

Comparability is important but it is only one part of the pay picture. We also need to look at the reasons why nurses' pay is so low, in order to develop a strategy which will avoid the constant struggle to maintain parity with other vaguely comparable groups — a struggle which has led to the depressingly familiar cycle of falling behind and catching up.

Women's work

The fact that nursing is still considered to be a female occupation has undoubtedly played a part in keeping wages low. Many women have always worked outside the home not just to earn 'pin money' but to provide necessary support for the family (especially if they are single parents) or to earn their own living, but it has always suited employers and

---

The two main approaches to nurses' pay

Professional organisations

- Nurses are a special case and deserve preferential treatment because they have failed to keep pace with other comparable skilled professionals.
- Nurses are trained, expert professionals and should be rewarded for that; untrained staff, i.e. auxiliaries and assistants, should not be included in such negotiations.
- Expertise and experience should be properly rewarded, and there should be incentives to stay in nursing created by maintaining the differentials between grades of staff — in other words, pay levels should reflect the hierarchical structure by ensuring that those at the top receive most, and so on down the scale. Such differentials can be maintained through percentage rises, which do not alter the relative levels of pay, and making minor adjustments to particular grades to evolve a satisfactory scale.
- The case can be won by reasoned argument, appeals to government decency, and pressure through such means as petitions, letter writing and public support.
- Industrial action cannot achieve its desired ends in a publicly funded non-profit-making service, and destroys public sympathy by breaking the nurse's bond of trust with her patients.

TUC trade unions

- The problem of nurses' low pay is shared by nearly all other workers in the NHS and all should fight together for improvements — unity is strength.
- All NHS workers, whether they are nurses, porters or cleaners, play a vital part in running the service and all deserve adequate recompense for their work.
- There is a place for differentials but they should not be maintained to the extent of failing to achieve significant improvements in the pay of those who fall below the government's own poverty line; this includes nursing auxiliaries.
- Appeals to public sympathy, petitions and so on may have some use but nothing substantial will be achieved without resort to more hard-hitting methods — meaning industrial action.
- Industrial action by health workers alone will not win the battle against low pay, partly because the effects of it harm those most in need, and not the employer. NHS workers must therefore enlist the support of more powerful workers in other industries.
- Pay campaigns should be part of an overall political, economic and social strategy which aims to secure justice and fair treatment for all.

governments to keep women's wages down by arguing that the money they earn goes to provide luxuries, not necessities.

In recent years the growing prominence of men in nursing has produced arguments that pay should be improved because the profession now contains more breadwinners and heads of families. It is tempting to use any argument that comes to hand in the search for more money, but this one should be avoided. Women are breadwinners and heads of families too and their time and labour is as valuable as the men's.

Discrimination against women, demonstrated in these arguments which attempt to deny them equality in the working world, is directly reflected in pay. Overall on average women earn only 60% of what men earn in similar jobs, and although the Equal Pay Act provided a legal framework to redress the balance, many employers have defied it or got round it by such devices as renaming women's jobs to avoid direct comparison with the men. Nursing does not face this problem directly but its place in the earnings scales suggests that its image as a women's job is still a relevant factor.

Service work

Women have traditionally tended to work in service jobs — often the only occupations open to them — and there is a direct link between this female labour force and the low values placed on such jobs. Cleaning, cooking and other domestic-type tasks are seen as an extension of women's natural sphere in the home and therefore not demanding or skilled enough to require much reward. Men's jobs like labouring or refuse collection are no more (or less) tiring or skilled, but receive better wages (although they are of course still relatively badly paid).

Nursing too is seen as a service job in some ways not far removed from domestic work, and this has influenced pay rates, or at least has given the employers an excuse for keeping wages low. It has also had the added burden of being regarded as a vocation — dedication, it is argued, should be its own reward — and pressure has been put on nurses not to complain, as this would display greedy self-seeking behaviour out of character with the 'service before self' ethic. Even today a few nurses argue that paying better wages would attract the 'wrong kind of girl' who would come into nursing for money and not for love.

Fortunately most nurses now reject such arguments and regard the improvements of their wages as a just reward for the energy and commitment they devote to their work. But the angelic image does serve to detract from an awareness of the expertise and effort the job involves, as opposed to the innate virtues of the caring nurse. This too may be a factor in the failure to secure better wages, since it is generally held that qualifications and inside knowledge and experience merit better pay, whereas dedication and instinctive skills do not.

Working in the public sector

Most nurses are employed by the NHS, and are therefore paid by public funds derived mainly from taxation. This has important consequences for pay. First, the amount of money allocated to the National Health Service, which varies according to the state of the economy and the political convictions of the government, directly governs the amount of money available for wage rises. In recent years the recession has led to increasingly tight control of the spending of public money, especially under Conservative governments which believe in restricting some public spending and encouraging private sector involvement in services such as health and education.

Nurses are the largest single group of workers in the NHS. Staff wages take up about 70% of the whole health service budget, and so the amount of money awarded to nurses in pay deals is crucial. When strict limits are placed on the money available to each health authority for wages and services, a high wage increase results in a shortage of funds for hospitals and other services, so attempts are obviously made to keep pay as low as possible. Nurses' wages account for a massive 40% of the whole NHS budget, and because they are so numerous, a large percentage rise in their pay means a huge increase in the total paybill — unlike, say, doctors, who can receive a substantial rise without hurting the budget too much because there are relatively few of them.

Another problem is the fact of working in an 'unproductive' job. In industry the workers may be able to point to such factors as increased profits in their claims for more money, but of course the Health Service makes no profit. Moreover, withdrawing your labour in the NHS simply saves public money and does not hit the employer where it usually hurts, in productivity and therefore profit — indeed, it can play into the hands of the private medical industry, which is only too pleased to profit from the shortcomings of the NHS. The state's virtual monopoly of health care is in sharp contrast to largely private systems like that in the

USA, where nurses are increasingly resorting to successful industrial action. As they are directly employed by private hospitals, withdrawing their labour affects the hospital's profitability and gives them a powerful weapon which can force substantial gains in a way impossible in the UK.

Nurses' pay is closely tied to the pay of all NHS workers, and in turn to public sector funding. NHS staff are among the lowest paid of all groups of workers, as a 1982 COHSE survey showed; almost half all full-time nursing staff earned a basic wage below the government's £82 a week poverty line. At a time when governments are keen to keep spending down by imposing ceilings on pay rises, public sector workers will be the hardest hit, because as government employees they are unavoidably subject to strict wage controls. Private sector workers have more hope of breaking through the recommended limit.

As the history shows, governments have resorted to calling special inquiries when dissatisfaction with low NHS pay becomes too great to ignore, usually resulting in reasonably large one-off rises. These have been particularly important to nurses, and helped to fuel discontent with the Whitley Council system of collective bargaining. It was no coincidence that the special awards followed periods of unrest in the NHS. Bodies like the RCN which oppose industrial action claimed that the special awards for nurses were the result of sustained pressure through reasoned argument and public and media campaigns, but the militancy of nurses at such times is also undoubtedly linked with the militancy of other NHS workers who are more willing to take industrial action. Some RCN nurses say their negotiators' hands are tied by the college's ban on strikes, though others feel it is a useful moral lever to apply to the government.

The longest dispute ever

In 1982 dissatisfaction with low pay and fears about the future of the NHS helped to produce the most sustained and severe disruption ever seen in the service (nearly a million working days were lost). Many nurses joined porters, ambulance crews and ancillary staff in days of protest, picket lines, working to rule and even withdrawing labour. These tactics were more effective than ever before because, for the first time, the different groups of NHS staff were all due for a rise on the same day, April 1st. This new common settlement date enabled the unions to call for action involving all groups of staff, rather than see them picked off and defeated one by one as each in turn was obliged to accept an unsatisfactory offer, as happened in previous disputes.

Nurses were more militant than ever before, but the traditional reluctance of most to take industrial action, and the important influence of the anti-strike RCN, led the government to try to divide them from the other NHS workers by offering them a slightly better rise. The Whitley Council staff side said this could be divided up to give most nurses an extra 6·4%, compared with 4% for most other groups. However, it was resoundingly rejected by their nurse members — by union nurses who did not want this special treatment, and by RCN members who thought the differential payment was derisory.

Despite its ban on strikes, the RCN found itself at the centre of the dispute — partly because it got off the mark very quickly with a campaign of petitions to MPs, protest rallies and letter writing, and partly because it held the balance of power on the Nurses and Midwives' Whitley Council. With the non-TUC staff organisations outnumbering the TUC affiliates by one seat, a decision by the RCN to accept or reject an offer could determine the final outcome. This time its members, on individual postal ballots, turned down the government's first two offers, to the delight and relief of the TUC unions. Acceptance by the nurses and midwives would destroy the NHS workers' united front, and indeed the dispute limped to an end after the RCN members accepted a third slightly improved offer.

Another factor in ending the dispute was the promise of a new review body to make recommendations on nurses' pay. Since 1980 desultory talks had been going on between the government, management and representative organisations to explore the possibility of a special arrangement to prevent nurses' pay falling behind that of other groups. This had made little progress because the government would not promise to fund any recommendations such a body might make, and because the TUC unions feared losing their powerful influence in the Whitley system. In the end, though, the promise proved to be the government's trump card. Fed up with disruptions to the service, anxious for more money in their pockets and hopeful that a new arrangement could be reached, nurses finally settled for a 12·3% rise spread over two years, and the promise of a new pay review body.

Bread today and jam tomorrow?

The new pay review body represents a far-reaching change in the way nurses' pay is determined, though it is doubtful whether it will produce the massive rises nurses feel they deserve. Until its establishment late in 1983, all staff in the NHS had their pay fixed through the collective bargaining machinery of the Whitley Councils, except for doctors and dentists who have a review body which was established in 1960. Now the pay of nursing staff, midwives and professions allied to medicine is decided by the government in the light of recommendations from an independent advisory panel. The body cannot increase the money available for nurses' wages, and may make it easier for the government to impose unpopular settlements — the representative organisations do not negotiate but simply present evidence. The new mechanism cannot make a significant difference unless more money comes from the Treasury, although ignoring any large recommendations it may make could put the government in an embarrassing position.

The most controversial issue surrounding the establishment of the review body was the decision whether to include in its remit unqualified staff such as nursing auxiliaries. The RCN, wanting recognition of the nurse's 'professional status' and hoping that smaller numbers of staff could secure larger rises, argued that, like the doctors and dentists' body, the review body should deal only with qualified nurses and midwives (adding, also, those in training — a concession to its strong student membership). The TUC unions, however, adamantly opposed the exclusion of auxiliaries, who comprise a large part of their nursing membership. In the event the government compromised: auxiliaries are included but the review body deals separately with qualified and unqualified nursing staff, and provides separate reports on nursing staff and the allied professions.

Further controversy surrounded the government's announcement that it reserved the right to exclude from the review body recommendations 'any groups that resort to industrial action' — claiming that the body was established in recognition of the refusal of most nurses to strike. This attempt to force on nurses an agreement not to strike was not mentioned publicly in the deal made to end the 1982 dispute, and continues the policy of driving a wedge between the professional organisations and TUC unions, whose cooperation could have been seriously damaging to the government in that dispute.

All in all the future is not particularly rosy for nurses' wage packets. The government has emphasised that however pressing the nurses' needs are, and however justified their claims, it is not bound to accept the review body's recommendations. It could refuse to do so for 'compelling national reasons'. The review body may be independent but it is purely advisory; continued pressure will be needed if nurses are to ensure that the government heeds its advice.

The moral to be drawn from this chequered history and its accompanying manoeuvrings is that nurses' pay, like everything else in nursing, cannot be properly understood in isolation from broader social and political concerns. The status of the job, the gender of the workers, economics and government policy all play their part. Moreover, the events also demonstrate the difficulty, impossibility even, of finding a single strategy to please all nurses. The disunity is often lamented, but it is unrealistic to expect so many people to agree on one approach. Pluralism may be uncomfortable and inconvenient but it is a fact of life, as well as a sign of healthy democracy.

Further Reading

Beale J. (1982). *Getting it together: women in trade unions*. London: Pluto Press.

Eaton J., Gill C. (1983). *The Trade Union Directory*. London: Pluto Press.

Gray A., Smail R. (1982). *Why has the nursing paybill increased?* Health Economics Research Unit discussion paper no. 01/82, University of Aberdeen.

Lancaster A. (1979). *Nursing and Midwifery Sourcebook*. London: George Allen & Unwin, *Nursing Times* Book Service edition.

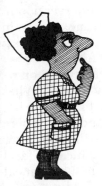

6

Where do we go from here?

Nursing and the NHS

Much of the discussion in this book has aimed to place nursing and nurses within the context of broader social, political and economic forces, based on the assumption that these forces largely determine who nurses are, the work they do, the way they do it and where they do it. Implicit in the discussion has been another assumption, that of a present and future in which health care is a collective social responsibility — reflected in the fact that health and social services are still mainly paid for by each citizen's contribution to central funds, resources then being redirected, in theory at least, to those most in need. Despite the current attacks on this principle, much discussion of nursing continues to be based on expectations that the major employer and major provider of education will continue to be the state.

The pattern of health care provision in a society which, at least nominally, offers services free at the point of delivery and makes some attempt to help disadvantaged groups — such as the poor, the old, the handicapped, the mentally ill — is discernibly different from one where services are tailored to meet the needs of those who can afford to pay directly for them. A comparison between the UK and the USA, for example, shows that our state-funded NHS offers far more in the way of community support and hospital care for those groups than the USA, where health care adheres more closely to the medical model of heroic intervention in disease. Comparing the systems is important not just from an ideological or moral standpoint, but because it also has major implications for nursing itself, and its future. As soon as the pole shifts from meeting needs to answering money-backed demands, other shifts immediately follow. What happens to nurse education and how is it funded? What about the unpopular fields such as mental handicap? Where does the professional power lie and whom is the consumer encouraged to trust (and pay)? How are education and service — or theory and practice — linked in a piecemeal system of independent, self-financing units? And so on.

In the UK nursing has been linked with state policy and funding for so long that we tend to forget the benefits it brings. Even today when the NHS is under threat, we assume that nursing policy and aims can be fed into statutory bodies and government departments which have the authority — given by consent — to direct the shape of things from the centre and to impose a uniform framework, and that our demands will get a hearing. How much flexibility there should be at local level is a matter of debate, but few challenge the need for some national norms or standards. Such assumptions have been made for many years, perhaps breeding complacency, so that nurses are often slow to acknowledge the interdependence of nursing and the NHS. More dangerously, many are also slow to come to the defence of threatened services and principles — possibly they do not realise how close to home such issues are. Only belatedly, when even establishment pillars like the British Medical Association are making a noise, have nurses as a group really begun to speak out against harmful government policies.

At the same time, much as many of us would like to plan nursing's future within the framework of the welfare state, and will fight tooth and nail to do so, it may also be sensible to take a realistic look at what is likely to happen in future. One straw in the wind was the UKCC's recent decision to become self-financing (mainly by making all qualified nurses fund it through periodic fees), a move largely caused by fears about the unreliability of central government funding and the potential it offers for interference in policy. Proposing that nurses should be professional workers who can offer their services on contract rather than as salaried employees has similar implications. Nurses should not rush headlong into assuming that central funding is gone for ever, and planning should be based on a hard-headed assessment of what is to come, but we must also consider how far such choices may help to hasten the demise of the welfare state and the NHS.

Another underlying theme of this book is the need to adapt nursing to changing patterns of care, so that the service we give and the way we are trained to give it matches the needs of the patient or client. This means flexible approaches to enable us to keep pace with moves to shift the care of mentally ill or handicapped people to the community, or to develop expertise in helping those with the problems of old age and chronic disability, to cite only two examples. The reasons why resources (and therefore interest, skills, research and education) are concentrated in particular areas are manifold and progress will be very difficult and slow — but nursing should lead the way in creating a service which is more responsive to need, rather than wait for doctors and governments to make the decisions. Of course this is not easy, but if we do not try, nursing will be at best a servant of other more powerful groups, and at worst a fossil.

Patterns of care are beginning to alter not only because of new perceptions and projections of need, but also because of changing public attitudes. People are less likely to take as gospel everything they are told by health professionals, and are seeking to know more and to be more actively involved in making the decisions which affect their lives. 'Consumer', the fashionable new word for the patient/client, is becoming popular because it carries the idea of a person who can pick and choose; like the customer in a shop, he or she can choose to withhold custom if the service is not satisfactory. This implies more independence and choice, but it also fits in with the private medical idea of customers and financial transactions; it is a less passive word than 'patient' but it still fails to put across the idea of 'partnership' now being proposed as a model for nurses/doctors/patients — working together for the ill or disabled person's well-being. Whatever label we use, however, the changing relationshps within and between health workers and users of services have major implications.

It is worth drawing together these threads, tangled and intertwined as they are, to summarise what we should bear in mind when planning change in nursing of any kind — in education, management, research or direct care-giving. Future health needs, the shrinking welfare state, the increase in (or reversion to) self care, all are contributing to a new world in which nursing must find its place — not only (as many desire) for reasons of occupational survival, but in order to determine how we can best contribute to people's well-being and how we can equip ourselves to do so.

Future needs

We have already seen that the national population profile is changing, with a declining birth rate and longer life expectancy, leading to a drop in the number of young people (itself significant for recruiting people to nursing) and a sharp increase in the proportion of elderly people, particularly those who are very old and frail. The decline in infectious diseases like TB and diphtheria, which used to be common killers, has enhanced the chances of survival, an epidemiological change which has come about through improved living standards and less poverty and deprivation. Medicine too has played a part in increasing the individual's chances of surviving a serious illness or accident; being born prematurely or with a major handicap is less likely to result in death. The overall picture is of a population generally healthier but with a greater proportion of old and handicapped people requiring support, and with greater inequalities in health between rich and poor.

There have also been changes in the prevalence and nature of disease. The decline in infectious diseases has been counterbalanced by the spread of other illnesses on an epidemic scale in the Western world, such as cancer or heart disease — often attributed to affluence, but like most other illnesses, bringing a higher death rate for people in lower social classes. This pattern of inequality has been fully documented in the Black report and elsewhere. Disease patterns are also changing in the psychiatric field, though it is hard to tell how far this is attributable to new definitions, new ways of classifying illness and new awareness of certain problems; the net result is fewer diagnoses of schizophrenia and more cases of alcoholism, drug dependency and short-term crises.

Generalisation on such a large scale is fraught with pitfalls, but it is widely acknowledged that the kinds of health problems which increasingly confront our health and social services include a vast number which are not amenable to medical intervention of the traditional kind (they may in fact never have been so, but the 'successes' of medicine have previously been unchallenged — like the claim to have eradicated infectious diseases). Frequently in general practice, for example, the doctor's appropriate response is counselling, support or advice rather than a prescription or referral to a specialist. Mental illness offers the challenge not of magic solutions through drugs or ECT, but of helping the sufferer to come to terms with the illness in the social context and to seek better health through changes in self, relationships and external circumstances. Disability, mental handicap and the problems of old age often call not for highly technical medicine or surgery but for practical help to live life as fully and independently as possible. Nursing may be slightly more attuned to such challenges than medicine, but both professions still have a long way to go in making their training, skills and interests match up to the requirements of those in need.

There is, too, a different philosophy abroad which stresses rehabilitation and the avoidance of over-long dependence on hospital care. Unfortunately this ties in readily with cost-cutting and it is sometimes hard to tell them apart: early discharge may be the preferred new mode of post-operative

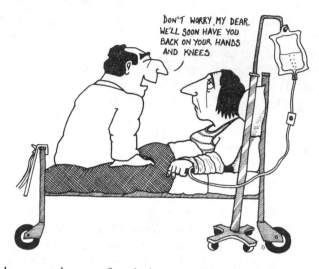

care but people are often being sent home long before they can cope. Day surgery is another option — on the increase — which avoids the dangers of too much hospitalisation and costs less, but again may not always be in the patient's best interests in the absence of well-staffed community services and other support networks. 'Care in the community' is not merely a government con and is certainly the pattern of the future, but the idea has been much abused by those looking for cheap alternatives to hospital provision. Good community care in fact is not cheap and requires considerable staff training as well as increased numbers.

The shrinking welfare state

Another cluster of factors we should not ignore in planning nursing for the future is the role of the state. This of course is closely linked to political questions and depends to some extent on the position of the elected government, but even under a Labour government with a much greater commitment to the welfare state, the squeeze would be likely to continue — not just in health care but in other major areas of public spending such as social services, benefits, education and housing. Cutbacks in all these fields have implications for health care, since they have knock-on effects on health, quite apart from the direct reduction in funds for employing and training health workers and providing facilities. In particular, removing the safety nets, inadequate as they often are, means many more people will fall below the poverty line — and poverty and ill health are closely linked, even in our relatively affluent society.

The groups which suffer most from welfare cuts are very often those who have more need of health care in the first place — such as people who are out of work and have a disability or mental illness, and the elderly, especially those who are frail or mentally ill. Other identified groups with health needs include people of ethnic minorities, who suffer from the racism of a monocultural health service, and newborn babies, who are twice as likely to die if they are born into a working class family. The talk about 'priority groups', adopted by both Labour and Conservative governments, has a major element missing, that of class inequalities in health — the gap between social classes in terms of health and expectations is actually widening. This too should be a priority, but it is treated with kid gloves because politically it is regarded as too hot to handle — or perhaps the solutions it points towards are too radical.

The shrinking welfare state therefore has implications not just for the future funding of health services and occupational training, but also for the general health of the population and the kinds of health care needs they are likely to have. The political shift to the centre is bringing with it an ideology of self-reliance, but many people are actually being deprived of the means of caring for themselves. For every scrounger there are many more people eking out a living on disability allowances or child benefits or old age pensions which are pathetically inadequate. Their need for health care is likely to grow rather than diminish, hospital admission often being their very last line of defence.

Discussion on these lines nearly always brings out the old 'bottomless pit' argument — that we only have finite resources to meet infinite demands. While it is true that spending the entire gross national product on health care would not solve every problem, the argument is really not a helpful one when we are seeking to solve the political and moral problems. There is no absolute line we can draw, but the decisions have to be made depending on how compassionate and civilised we want our society to be. And even given those finite resources, there is a great deal more we can do to ensure that they are spent in the most equitable way and on those who really need it most. The 'bottomless pit' is usually a smokescreen thrown up to avoid the real politics involved, and also to deflect attention from the fact that political systems and the use of resources depend on power and not on some 'natural' state of things.

Self care

The idea of self care has some worthy origins in a genuine belief that recovery from illness or coping with disability starts with the patient, and that the health professional cannot and should not assume control of that person's life. What they can do is help them along the way by teaching them how to help themselves — a philosophy which is applicable in far more health care settings than is often appreciated. Even someone undergoing major surgery very quickly returns to a state where they can exercise considerable autonomy. The growing acceptance of the idea of partnership between patient and professional is demonstrated in the latest nursing care and teaching, a trend which as we have seen ties in with more vocal consumers and the challenge to professional domination in many fields, not just medicine.

Unfortunately, as we have seen, the helpful and caring aspects of the idea of self care are being given a bad name by the government. 'Self care' is being imposed on all sorts of people without the necessary back-up — the philosophy provides window dressing for the move away from collective social responsibility for the weaker, poorer or otherwise disadvantaged members of our society. But either way the trend is probably here to stay, and is one which should be taken into account in nursing.

The pressing problem now facing nursing is that of finding

a place in this changing landscape. We are likely to see a smaller number of well-equipped hospitals offering the latest technology and medical developments (some of them privately owned); some long-stay hospitals, but much more primary and community care; and all this in the context of different assumptions about who gives the care and how they should be prepared. Paradoxically we can perhaps see these changes most clearly in fields like mental handicap, precisely because they are at the bottom of the heap and have the least to lose, and the least interference from the power groups; and perhaps it is no coincidence that the greatest challenge to nurses to prove that they are indeed the most appropriate and best prepared care givers has come in mental handicap. The response should not be to defend nursing to the death, but to look clearly and dispassionately at the needs of the people and then to decide how best these needs can be met. If nurses cannot do this, they may face the same fate as the dinosaur — which failed to adapt, and paid the penalty.

The picture today

These, then, are some of the trends which will help to determine the future of nursing as an occupation. How do they fit in with the reality of giving nursing care today, in hospital or community? A major aim of this book has been to look at the comments and strategies of the government, senior nurses and leaders of the profession in the light of what really happens at the 'coalface', and it has been striking to see that reality is often ignored in the pursuit of particular goals. More and more people are working hard to close the gap, in different fields and in different organisations, but there is still a sense that many of these decision-makers are living in another world far removed from the daily concerns of ordinary people, whether staff or patients.

Value for money

No nurse can have failed to notice the government's latest war cry, 'value for money'. The boom years are past, we are told, and everyone must tighten their belts — including public services like the NHS which are supposed to have been rolling in clover. Efficiency savings are the order of the day; health authorities are establishing value for money committees (already, in true health service fashion, abbreviated to VFM — a sign of how freely the phrase has passed into the jargon). These scrutinise areas of spending previously immune from such inspection, while strict cash limits are being imposed to ensure that spending stays within the government's targets.

In spite of government claims that the budget cuts were intended only to 'trim the fat' and would not affect patient care, 1983 saw the imposition of strict new manpower targets which resulted in reductions in the previously sacrosanct 'front line' jobs of medicine and nursing. These cuts, moreover, were made not in the establishment but in the numbers of staff actually in post on March 31, meaning all vacancies disappeared at a stroke. Staffing levels have also been reduced in jobs which provide essential back-up services, such as porters and domestics, thus creating extra workloads for nurses who as usual fill in the gaps. The favourite Tory target of 'bureaucracy' has led to a smaller number of ward clerks and other clerical staff, for example, making the health service less rather than more efficient and diverting clinical staff from their time spent with patients.

Privatisation, the policy of inviting outside contractors to run services such as laundry and catering which were previously run in-house, has also had knock-on effects for nurses, quite apart from the unjust treatment of low paid workers who are being re-employed by the contractors at lower wages and with fewer benefits. In general health authorities have bowed extremely reluctantly to government pressure on this, and it is early days, but there are suggestions that standards decline when cost-cutting private companies are brought in — again passing a bigger workload on to the ward nurse, who has to make good the deficiencies when cleaning is not done often enough or the washing up is not finished.

The less obvious effects of the health spending squeeze

include the deteriorating conditions of many hospitals and clinics, making the environment less safe for both patients and staff, with a moratorium on much new building. Health and safety hazards multiply when old plant is not replaced and staff make do with obsolete equipment, yet health service premises, as Crown property, are immune from prosecution under the Health and Safety at Work Act. Facilities for staff are often primitive and the meals in hospital canteens break all the rules of good nutrition laid down by the DHSS itself. Nurses are having to wash their own uniforms and live in residences which are more like a barracks than a home — and even these are being sold off to private buyers.

More hidden cuts are affecting the quality of education and training, especially in the post-basic area. Cost-conscious authorities are increasingly reluctant to give nurses study leave or pay for them to attend courses, preventing them from developing their professional knowledge and their careers. Schools and colleges have less money to buy textbooks and the quality of education in the clinical areas suffers when the workload is too great to permit teaching and supervised practice.

Senior nurses have been slow to speak up on this appalling state of affairs. They seem reluctant to acknowledge what is really happening on the wards and in the community, and are placed in the ambivalent position of having to implement cuts with which they might disagree — the sheer size of the nursing budget attracts unwelcome attentions. New changes in the management structure are jeopardising many of their jobs, another reason to remain silent. When the chief nurse of a London health authority, who also happened to hold a senior post in the RCN, publicly protested at cutbacks in his district, he was hailed as someone with exceptional courage, even though others more junior had been saying the same thing for several years. The TUC unions' constant protests had already become a regular ritual before the RCN finally entered the lists with its 'Nurse Alert' campaign, leading up to the publication of a new pamphlet documenting the effects of the cuts.

These comments were sent to the Royal College of Nursing after its call for evidence on the effects of NHS cuts.

'Last month while I was on annual leave the staffing levels were very low. For example, on one morning shift a third year student nurse was in charge, a first year nurse and second year nurse and one auxiliary completed the team. That morning there were seven operations, four admissions and four discharges. How can patients be adequately nursed? How can student and pupil nurses be supported with such staffing levels? I have very little job satisfaction at the moment. The only encouragement I have is the gratitude from most patients and the continued enthusiasm from student and pupil nurses. I continue to be amazed that they battle on and cope — but for how long can they take such stress and responsibility?'

Ward sister, London.

'It is becoming impossible to be at the bedside and get to know the patients under our care and for whom we are ultimately responsible. Less and less time is available to supervise and teach the student nurses yet new methods are being introduced — for example, the nursing process. Patients are at risk.'

SRN, Kent.

'This district is very deprived. There are only 33 mental illness beds for a population of 282 000 and minimal psychogeriatric beds. There may be capital resources but the limited manpower is going to affect the plans to move staff from the acute sector to the priority and community areas.'

District nursing officer, Trent region.

Extracts taken from the *Nurse Alert* report, available from the publications department, Royal College of Nursing, 20 Cavendish Square, London W1M 0AB.

Nurse Alert was criticised for being too anecdotal, but there is no doubt that the strength of feeling it expressed is shared by many nurses throughout the country. It also encouraged the RCN's leaders to make strong public statements deploring the cuts. Much of the material echoed nurses' comments dating back at least seven or eight years — my own cuttings collection contains many examples. But as the chorus of protest has grown, so has the government's resolve, boosted by Margaret Thatcher's re-election in May 1983. Now it is implementing a new managerial plan which will give even greater financial control and executive authority to a single general manager in each authority and even in each unit of management (such as a hospital or group of specialist or community services). At one stroke this plan, recommended to the government after an inquiry carried out by Roy Griffiths, the managing director of Sainsbury's, will destroy the system of consensus management whereby each member of the multidisciplinary team could contribute directly to decision-making; now the power will be held by a single person, usually a lay administrator and usually a man. Some management teams have barely established themselves since the last NHS reorganisation, but must now undergo yet another major upheaval.

The nursing reaction to this scheme has tended to dwell on the real or supposed snub to nurse managers contained in the Griffiths report, which suggested by implication or omission that they were inefficient and ineffective. Now areas such as staffing and personnel, and above all, budgetary control, will no longer be run by nurses, whose role in senior management and planning will in the main be reduced to an advisory one. Unfortunately the senior nurses found their voice too late; moreover their protests dwelt too much on their own loss of power and not enough on the broader political implications of 'Griffiths'. Now ministers have appointed a businessman with no knowledge of health care to the post of NHS general manager, moreover a man with a track record of involvement in privatising nationally owned resources. The emphasis will lie even more firmly on industrial-style management with all the associated ideas of productivity, efficiency and the consequent financial restraints, which have little to do with the quality of health care and a lot to do with cutting costs.

This is not to claim that the NHS is already highly efficient (though the proportion of its budget spent on administration is the lowest in the West) and that there is not room for much improvement; Griffiths' emphasis on consumer satisfaction also has much to commend it. But these proposed improvements are window dressing to the main aim of cutting costs.

Resources and priorities

Arguments about the cuts are often met with comments that the crisis is not new, and that complaints about shortages have been made since the NHS was first established in 1948. But whether the crisis is new or constant, it is serious, especially for those people who depend on health care for their very existence and yet who cannot speak out on their own behalf. As we have seen, the acute services have always carried off the lion's share of the budget, and despite claims that priorities have shifted to the deprived areas, in terms of both specialties and geographical districts, little has changed. The cost comparisons show that chronic, long-stay, mental illness and mental handicap hospitals receive only a fraction of the money spent on acute hospitals: calculated on a basis of the cost per in-patient week in each type of hospital, the bottom line is the mental handicap hospitals, which have far less to spend per patient not just on medical or nursing skills, but on catering, cleaning and domestic needs — yet for many residents these hospitals are their only home.

Indeed, events in the last few years suggested not a shift to under-resourced areas but just the opposite — a tendency to shield the prestigious acute hospitals, especially the teaching hospitals, from the cuts; many smaller local hospitals have been closed as 'uneconomic' while the district general hospital emerged relatively unscathed. Yet even this immunity is disappearing, with major bed closures at world famous hospitals showing that no-one is now safe from the axe (the

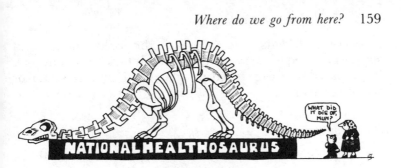

nearby presence of private medical developments, inciden-
tally, being more than coincidence). Five years ago it would
have been hard to believe that whole wards would close at a
hospital like Guy's, but it has happened. Funds are being
diverted, it is claimed, to poorer areas of the country but the
crudity of resource allocation formulas means Peter is
robbed to pay Paul, and growth is at a standstill, so everyone
ends up worse off.

The 'community' is held to be another priority area, yet it
claims only around 10% of the budget even though most
people's contact with the health service is through their
general practitioner, contraception clinic, health visitor or
school health service. Within the priority areas, resources
are supposed to be moved from hospital to community,
enabling many more mentally ill, mentally handicapped and
old people to lead more normal lives in the mainstream of
society, yet the staff fear that the closure of the large hospitals
and the profitable sales of the grounds will not necessarily
liberate new funds for the new developments — a justifiable
scepticism in the light of this government's record. Mean-
while early discharge, greater patient turnover and social
service cuts are putting more burdens on community nurses
who are already hard pressed. Some hospitals are discharg-
ing patients to 'the community' in the shape of privately run
hostels and nursing homes where sometimes the residents
are exploited and even locked out from morning till night. It
is vital to ensure that patients are prepared properly for their
move to the outside world and that efforts are made to
provide the right help and accommodation, but too often
'community care' amounts to forcing responsibility on

relatives or friends who may lack the skills, money and support needed to carry out this difficult task, or to dumping ill-prepared and frightened people on the private sector or social services.

Private medicine

Nursing homes and hostels of the type mentioned above have long been the backbone of the UK's private health sector, often providing facilities which the state will not, and often giving good care to the elderly and the disabled. Some homes in this independent sector are run by charities and voluntary organisations and again standards may be high. But now the unsung efforts of such people are being over-shadowed and to some extent tainted by the boom in the private medicine market, for speculators have not been slow to move in where the government was happy to find an opening and shift responsibility from the public to the private purse. Property developers are busy buying up large houses, old hotels or former NHS premises to sell as potential nursing homes or private hospitals.

The growth in this area, where private companies move in to take care of elderly, mentally ill or disabled people who can afford to pay, or whose relatives can, may prove to be more significant than the highly publicised developments in acute private medicine. There are in fact signs that the boom in acute private medicine during the late 1970s and early 1980s has reached a plateau, for some of the hospitals built to cream off paying patients in middle-class areas have failed to attract a high enough turnover, while the growth in the uptake of private health insurance — essential for the growth of private acute services, since few people can afford the services without it — is also falling off. Paybeds in NHS hospitals and the glossy, hi-tech, American-style facilities advertised nationally have so far been the chief focus of trade union and Labour opposition, but this acute sector may by its very nature only ever cater for a small fraction of the population. Important as this is, the less heralded growth in private care for long-stay patients may prove to be more of a threat to the NHS, since it appears to provide an alternative to services which enjoy little public affection or support and gives the government an excuse to cut them back even further.

Although the Tories' original claim that the private/ independent sector could eventually be responsible for 25% of the UK's health care now seems unlikely, or at least premature, their determination to enable it to cash in on the NHS has worrying implications for nurses and for the future of state health care. By offering the image of an attractive, de luxe alternative, the acute private sector undermines public support for the NHS, offering a model of health care which suggests that illness can be cured by expensive medical or surgical intervention, even though it relies on NHS-trained staff and NHS back-up facilities and will not provide care which does not make profits.

The fact that one private company, Private HealthCare Ltd., was prepared to advertise itself through favourable comparisons with the NHS ('When you're old, the last place you want to be is in hospital', under a crude cartoon of a scruffy NHS geriatric ward) shows that the private sector is trying to compete by luring people away from the NHS, whatever the talk of 'partnership', and by implying that the NHS offers a second class service. Its approach reinforces the view that good health is about what goes on between doctor and patient, and ignores the broader implications of health policy, recognition of the social causes of ill health and the factors which aid recovery and rehabilitation. The Tories, like the acute private sector, would like us to see ill health and the ability to pay for health care as a personal problem. Private care takes us even further away from the idea of collective responsibility, and the possibility of collective solutions to health problems. It also undermines the coherent local planning and provision of a full range of services.

The implications are great for nurse training and staffing. The private sector makes virtually no contribution to basic nurse training and offers very little in the way of post-basic, in-service or specialist education, but it is happy to employ people who have gained skills in the NHS, and in most cases pays them the same or lower wages (sometimes without the terms and conditions of service imposed on the NHS by the Whitley Councils, putting the nurse at a disadvantage). Areas with a large concentration of private beds, such as inner London, recruit staff badly needed in NHS hospitals. Trade union membership is discouraged or forbidden but RCN membership is allowed or even paid for by the employer; the indemnity insurance for RCN members means the company would not have to pay for a nurse's negligence if she were sued for damages.

The private sector may as yet be marginal in the acute area, if not in the twilight zone of nursing homes for the elderly, but it has great ideological importance, which is why it has become a battleground. While it is undoubtedly a threat to socialised health care, there is also much nurses can learn from it, for it feeds on legitimate dissatisfactions with the NHS — especially in the area of personal relations and respect for the patient. It is in the private hospital's interest to treat its clients as though they were all oil-rich sheiks, since their future custom is important, and clearly many people are prepared to pay through the nose for the personal touch which is often sadly lacking in the NHS.

'Efficiency savings', cuts, unjust resource allocation, and private medicine all have a profound effect on today's health services, both the quality of the care given and the satisfaction of staff and patients. In particular all have profound effects on nursing too. Travelling down the road offered by the government and big business suggests a future for nursing in technical medical care with a concentration of skills in the acute sector, following medicine's lead rather than looking at people's health needs, moving away from a comprehensive education system for health staff, and leaving unpopular client groups to be cared for mainly by auxiliaries and families with few resources and no support. Is this really where we want to go?

Nursing under stress

Things are not looking good for the poor old NHS. But how is the individual nurse faring amid all these problems? As part of the only group of people in direct contact with patients round the clock, she really is working at the sharp end, experiencing the effects of these policies and attempting to make good their deficiencies. What of her own personal survival?

It should already be clear from this book that nurses are keeping the service going only at great personal cost. People going into a badly paid job like nursing and knowing they will work very hard on unsociable shifts may have low expectations, but even so there are many signs that nurses, traditionally uncomplaining and self-effacing people, are finding it hard to keep going. The nursing press, conferences and study days are paying increasing attention to subjects like stress and 'burnout', the syndrome which results from prolonged exposure to stress at work; now that the nursing culture is becoming a little more humane and relaxed, such a debate is more acceptable and many nurses are for the first time finding they have enough support to be able to express their feelings of stress and anxiety. To some degree the problems may always have been there, but now they are coming into the daylight and demanding attention.

There are many different definitions of stress and it is by nature difficult to pin down or measure. Something which stresses one person may excite another, and certainly a life with no stresses would be dull; stress may be stimulating, make you feel more alive and encourage personal growth through crisis. But it certainly seems that too much of it is definitely not a good thing, and the evidence we have suggests that nursing is a job which places a great deal of stress on individuals. Much of the evidence is inevitably anecdotal, but it is none the less persuasive or important for that, and it is not hard to find — talk to any nurse for long enough and it will emerge. Other measures of stress include absenteeism, sickness, drop-out rates from training, and the number of qualified nurses who never return to the occupation. Factors other than stress are involved, but it is surely a major reason, as indicated in the few studies and in anecdotal evidence. The statutory body reports a growing number of nurses coming before its professional conduct committee with problems related to drink and drug abuse, another sign that all is not well.

Some of the factors behind these high levels of stress and its many casualties — discussed elsewhere in this book — include the nature of the work, the repressive and hierarchical nursing system, the high demands and expectations of many patients, the lack of support and the individualisation of problems. Add to that low pay, unsociable hours, shift work, poor facilities and discourteous or even unpleasant treatment from seniors and doctors, and it is surprising that anyone stays in nursing at all. On top of all that there is the perennial resource crisis and the latest attacks on the NHS, all serving to give the nurse more work with less staff and fewer resources. Through it all, nurses grit their teeth and carry on, trying to prove to the world, each other and themselves that they can 'cope'.

Such determination may in some ways be admirable, but it also masks a reluctance, perhaps born of fear, to admit the truth about the conditions of the job. Stress in nursing is taking a heavy toll not only of students and junior grades, but of senior nurses: Hingley's survey showed that 42% of the 650 senior nurses sampled were under strain from feelings of inadequacy and isolation at work. All the evidence suggests a great sea of unhappiness, or an iceberg whose tip appears in wastage rates or professional conduct committees but whose bulk is unseen and largely unheeded. On humanitarian grounds alone the problem must be tackled. How can we presume to care for others without caring for the people who do the job?

There are other compelling reasons for looking for solutions to the stress epidemic, though they are less important than the need to prevent misery. Economically it makes poor sense to run a service where people are constantly dropping out, going off sick or leaving as soon as they qualify, and moreover the quality of the care is affected when morale is low. Depressed and overworked nurses are hardly in a position to nourish and support their patients. In the future nursing may appear an unattractive option — and with the pool of potential recruits under the age of 20 shrinking dramatically, we cannot for much longer afford to force people out by failing to look after them in the way they are told to look after others.

In many ways nurses are the victim of being part of a large labour force with a very high turnover. There are simply so many nurses, and so many of them changing jobs or ward placements so often, that they are treated as expendable, since for every one who drops out or disappears another always comes to take her place. It is hard to get across the message that the problem is a collective and not an individual one, although some individualised responses to tackling stress can be extremely helpful. The problems are experienced individually and pressure is felt by the individual nurse, rather than nurses as a group. Yet to achieve widespread success in fighting stress and indeed in preventing it, we must learn to think and act together. This does not mean smothering disagreement, but it does mean taking responsibility together, acknowledging the shortcomings of the system and trying to change it, being alive to each other's needs and ensuring that we evolve good mechanisms for support and prevention. This starts with the acceptance that the nurse who suffers the ill effects of stress is not a weak, feckless, unsuitable or irresponsible individual, but the victim of a largely uncaring and unthinking system. To alleviate stress in nursing we have to change that system, and start by changing it from within.

Individualism — the answer?

A number of practical suggestions have been made to help the nurse avoid or deal with stress and its effects in a constructive and self-enhancing way. As long ago as 1972 the Briggs committee saw the establishment of nurse counsellors as an urgent priority, yet there is still only a handful of full-time counsellors working in the nursing setting, and even this slow progress seems to be regarded by some as a luxury (compare this with further/higher education, where student counsellors are the norm). Others view counselling services with suspicion because the word is too often used as a synonym for discipline; nurses coming back from sick leave may be sent to a senior nurse for 'counselling', in other words interrogation about why they were ill. Yet the first rule of true counselling is that it should be offered by someone who is independent of management, school or any other power structure, and that it should be the client's choice to participate. Neither is it a fancy word for a chat over a cup of tea, for the counsellor must be properly trained and able to deal with the difficulties and strong feelings which may emerge.

It is a pity that the abuse of it should give counselling a bad name, for it undoubtedly achieves an enormous amount in settings where it is offered by a skilled practitioner. Some managers and tutors unfortunately use such a service as a way of passing the buck, and there should be no excuse for failing to treat juniors in a humane and supportive manner just because there is a counsellor as a safety net. On the whole, though, the existence of a good service seems to encourage a feeling that counselling is valid and helpful, and may help to transform the hospital or clinic into a more caring environment. Where staff refer themselves instead of being sent, the uptake of the service can be quite high, which not only shows the level of need but suggests that the service quickly loses any stigma associated with being only for the mad or the bad. Nurse tutors often regard themselves as counsellors and have a vital part to play in giving the student warmth, encouragement, sympathy and support. But again their role should not be confused with that of a trained counsellor, whose relationship with the student is not complicated by hierarchical or disciplinary power. However, so few senior nurses have seen fit to introduce a counselling service that there is a shortage of evidence on it in the nursing field, and a lack of word-of-mouth experience which could encourage more to take the plunge.

At best counselling can develop the individual nurse's strength and self-esteem, encouraging her not to internalise the difficulties of her work or blame herself for everything. It may also give her the confidence to challenge some of the abuses she experiences and to hand the responsibility back where it belongs. Similar results can be achieved through the different but related area of assertiveness training, which is becoming talked about quite extensively in nursing and being introduced into some basic training programmes. Anne Dickson, a psychologist who is largely responsible for introducing and developing assertiveness training in the UK, defines it as the art of clear, honest, direct communication. This may sound simple but it depends on a foundation of high regard for yourself and for others, the former in particular being an attribute many nurses do not share, for most are women brought up to subordinate their needs to others — a condition which is reinforced by nursing training and its ethic of self-effacing dedication.

As a practical method of dealing with stress, assertiveness training has much to recommend it. By encouraging assertive rather than passive or aggressive behaviour, and teaching it through specific behavioural exercises, it helps the nurse to cope more effectively with the demands made on her, often by giving her the ability and strength to draw the line, to say no and not to feel guilty if she chooses not to comply with every request. The techniques not only help the individual nurse to reduce her own stress, but may transform her working environment through a change in atmosphere and the way in which problems are tackled.

Being assertive is part of good communications and it is probably no coincidence that the techniques are being used in some schools of psychiatric nursing, since communication is of paramount importance there and is increasingly recognised as such. That realisation is slowly spreading too to the general field, and there is now an extensive literature on the subject, with 'communication skills' appearing on more and more curricula. Here the emphasis is on the nurse/patient interaction, however, rather than on the nurse herself in relation to others and her work. In the same way counselling is stressed not only as a tool to help her, but as a skill she should incorporate in her practice to become a better nurse. Articles on the nurse as counsellor and communicator often start by berating nurses for their shortcomings in these areas, and carry strong overtones of expectation that the nurse must be a superhuman being whose own needs and problems simply have no place in her work. There is also a sense that the patient is a passive recipient of the nurse's communications and that s/he too is expected to behave in a model way (causing no disruption, being reasonable and unemotional, certainly not being 'difficult'). As Angie Cotter pointed out, in the *Medicine in Society* articles on nursing, the advice also tends to skate over or ignore the larger issues which act as communication blocks, whether they are of an institutional or more personal kind.

Counselling and communication are issues which concern both the nurse-as-person and the nurse-as-worker, two aspects which tend to be viewed and treated separately but which are in truth interdependent, parts of the same whole and heavily influenced by each other. The same is true of other preoccupations such as the nursing process and holistic patient care, but here the nurse disappears from view altogether as a person and exists only in relation to the patient. As we shall see, such ideas contain much that is valuable and creative, but like so much else in nursing they are often talked about in isolation from context (or else the context is introduced as a sub-section on a nursing history form, to be charted and then filed away and forgotten).

Whatever is good and valuable in these new ideas, the form in which they are expressed tends to place yet more responsibility on the individual nurse — just like the popular notion of accountability. In typical nursing fashion, problems are identified and nurses are then blamed for not sorting them out, for failing to meet patients' needs, for being haphazard and unsystematic in their care, for fragmenting the whole person, for a whole multitude of shortcomings. The critique may sometimes be justified but it is rarely made in the context of looking at the real conditions in which nurses work and the real difficulties they face in keeping the service together, let alone in being counsellors, communicators, record-keepers, spiritual guides, skilled technicians, and so on and on. It is not just reactionary resistance to change of any kind which has caused the nursing process to founder on the rocks of indifference, but a justifiable reluctance to adopt new methods which not only appear to create more work but also put the blame for failure at the individual's door — and give her greater responsibility without any corresponding support, understanding or reward.

This is all demonstrative of the individualism of the nursing culture. Problems, and solutions, are laid at the individual's door, and there is a refusal to tackle problems collectively or in a social context. Individual answers are sought without changing the basis of the system which creates many of the problems in the first place. All this means more pressure on the nurse rather than less; so far the solutions we have found, even the most radical, tend to be ways of controlling rather than solving or preventing problems. Such solutions do have their place, but without collective action and collective responsibility they will at best be only partially successful, and may even sometimes be positively harmful.

Hope for the future

The picture I have painted so far is a gloomy one, and I believe rightly so. But the future need not be so gloomy if nurses can make full use of their potential to adapt and even transform the care they give in order to meet tomorrow's needs. By doing so we will be helping to stem the tide of callousness, greed and exploitation which threatens to engulf so many of the advances this country has made towards a more humane and caring society. We cannot do it alone, but within the health care system there are great possibilities if we can learn how to use them.

First there is the sheer weight of numbers of nurses. Although as a group and as individuals nurses are not regarded as powerful or influential, and there are forces at work to prevent them from being so, the potential is there. Imagine the power for change if nurses decided to act together, to introduce new ways of giving health care or to oppose a particular policy! So far we have lacked the unity and the organisation, but we might have more courage if we remembered that nurses numerically are by far the largest occupational group in the NHS. If three quarters of a million people agreed to act together, the results could be astounding.

Not only are we strong in numbers, we have as potential allies the people who are the reason for our existence as nurses — the patients and clients. Nurses have the closest contact with them and know most about their needs; the current popularity of the idea of the nurse as patient advocate suggests the possibility of alliance. This closeness is essential in providing good care in the broadest sense, for only by being aware of each person's health needs through close contact can the care and treatment given be appropriate. This contact is something we have now and could develop more strongly, but we risk losing it in the blind pursuit of professionalism along medical lines, which — as doctors demonstrate — tends to create divisions between people rather than bring them together. Indeed the medical establishment and its ideals and methods of practice is probably the single biggest barrier to change; to ally ourselves with medicine and the curative model of intervention through power, rather than the caring model which emphasises partnership and social context, is to side with the powerful and not the powerless and with reaction and not progress.

The nurse often holds a key role in relation to other health workers, as the pivot of the team in the day-to-day organisation of care if not in the hierarchy of power and influence. Here too she has great potential to be a guide and guardian of true teamwork, another essential aspect of the best model of future health care. Just as the patient's needs cover a wide spectrum, so do the workers who help to satisfy them, whether it is the cooks, the laundry workers or the ancillaries who wash their lockers. And it is the nurse who is best placed to facilitate and promote good caring relationships between the staff as well as with the patients. The ward sister in particular sets the style or tone of the ward and can do enormous good (or harm) in creating good teamwork — meaning the whole team and not just the 'professional' members usually implied in the idea.

Rather than allying ourselves with medicine, then, nurses

can help to create better relationships throughout the health care system — a role for which we are well suited partly through the nature of our work, but also through gender and class. To some extent the desire to link up with medicine reflects aspirations to be middle class, but this desire, and the obstacles erected in some nursing schools to exclude working class or black students, ignore the fact that most patients are not middle class and feel more at home in a strange or frightening situation with someone whose speech and behaviour is more familiar to them — again an important way of developing the vital bond with patients which leads to satisfaction of their needs.

For similar reasons the predominance of women in nursing should be seen as a strength and not a weakness. The influx of men into nursing is said to bring higher status, more political dynamism and so on, but the advantages to patients of having female nurses are rarely mentioned. It may be the result of conditioning, but clearly many people of both sexes find it easier to talk intimately to a woman than to a man. Research shows that women are better listeners, less likely to interrupt and interpose their own needs or ideas, and less inhibited about accepting emotion in others and allowing them to express feelings freely without embarrassment. This concern for others can lead and has led to exploitation of women but it is also a great and valuable strength, and one of which nurses seem sadly unaware, sharing as they do the generally low valuation of women's caring qualities.

This is not female chauvinism. Men in nursing may also demonstrate such qualities, and it is not necessarily an argument for maintaining a majority of women in nursing. But given that doctors, even female ones, tend to represent the hard scientific edge of health care — remote, detached, disinterested, technically competent — the nurse should cling even more closely to those warm humanitarian qualities on which the patient depends so heavily. And to do that means valuing our attributes as women, rather than doing ourselves down or feeling that masculine medical attributes and skills are more important. Nurses/women should realise that doctors/men have much to learn from them.

Nursing's other enormous strength is its ability to adapt to changing needs and patterns of care. Although we have tended to be hidebound by tradition, we do through our statutory bodies control our training, and we are the people who give most of the care; what is to stop us transforming our practice in the ways we think most appropriate? If the doctors make a fuss, well, we have the strength to argue our case. Make a fuss they certainly will, and have already. While negotiation with them is important, and preferable to confrontation, we should do this from a position of strength and a firm belief in our own rightness. It is they who are out of time; the model we propose will be a lot more relevant to health care in the 21st century. Already within nursing we possess a huge range of skills and experience of working in different settings — if we truly share this and learn from each other, we will be well equipped for the future challenges, much more so than the doctors, who are on the whole trained only to cure sickness and not to rehabilitate or support or promote good health.

Nursing therefore has many strengths, and perhaps all we need to learn is how to harness them. Subverting medical domination, a goal to be sought not for occupational imperialism and self-seeking, but because it is necessary for our patients' well-being, can be done in many ways other than a head-on clash with the medical establishment. Primarily we must ally ourselves with patients, continuing to speak their language and promote their interests; every day this can be done in hundreds of apparently small ways. Promoting health and preventing illness, fighting politically to end the social causation of ill health, bridging the professional gap in a real partnership with patients, and choosing people before technology; this adds up to a compelling new charter for nursing.

Good practice

Happily there are signs that such an alliance is beginning to emerge in nursing, although it is a slow process and many vested interests oppose it. New philosophies of care, if they are not enacted with due support and concern for the carers, can become another kind of oppression for the nurse at the sharp end, and those who are introducing change most successfully are those who have the highest regard for the people doing the work (often, of course, they are doing it themselves rather than preaching from a distance). The nursing process or the use of research findings can become more sticks with which to beat the nurse and to underline her shortcomings. There are many examples of good practice, and a growing sensitivity to individual needs, which manage to introduce new approaches in a realistic way, but constant vigilance is needed to make sure the spirit of the innovation is kept alive. The introduction by force of a care pattern which purports to be based on individual choice and meeting needs is a contradiction which hardly provides a good role model or encourages people to change. It puts into question the original motives for the change — is it merely jumping on a bandwagon, or using jargon or a pseudoscientific mystique to raise the status of the occupation? It is not just the ideas that count, but the way they are put into practice — and this is often very revealing of the philosophy behind the window dressing.

The growing recognition that each patient is an individual with specific wants and needs — how extraordinary that this should ever have been forgotten! — is at the root of many exciting and promising new developments in the clinical and educational fields. For example, the nursing process is no more than an instrument or a means to achieve certain goals, but it does encourage systematic assessment of a patient's needs, rational planning of care and evaluation of its effectiveness — a simple, logical approach which discourages performing tasks automatically because they have always been done, regardless of their value. Above all it should place the patient at the centre of events, rather than being one of a production line, and when properly used can encourage the nurse to have a much more sensitive awareness of individual needs and specific solutions to problems.

The conceptual approach underlying the process of nursing suggests a model of care which is far removed from the medical one of disease diagnosis–treatment–cure. Instead it suggests moving from assessment of ability to carry out the normal activities of life, through help and support, towards self care and independence — a much more creative way of looking at healing as a cycle of events with the person in need as the focus, instead of the disease or problem he or she presents. Clearly this is a much more sensible and fruitful approach, too, in view of the types of health problems people have and the enormous need for support and rehabilitation within the priority groups of the old, the mentally ill, the mentally handicapped and the disabled. Even in acute settings where the care is more medically oriented, it makes a lot more sense to encourage individual development and participation in the progress to recovery. Such an approach emphasises the patient's strengths rather than weaknesses, avoids domination by a professional practitioner and offers much more potential for personal involvement and creative input on the patient's part — an active rather than passive role.

One of the most promising ways of using the nursing process is being developed by Roper, Logan and Tierney, three British nurses who have evolved a model for nursing as a framework for nursing practice. It incorporates the process steps of assessment, planning, intervention and evaluation, and focuses on the individual patient's activities of living, thus helping the nurse and patient to identify problems in each specific area, to set goals and carry through the other steps of the process. In itself the model appears practical, sensible — common sense, indeed — and easily understood, all crucial if it is to cut any ice with the busy nurse. Moreover the authors have taken great care to work with nurses using the model in different settings and to modify their conclusions in the light of experience. Unlike many nursing theorists, they have the courage to link theory and practice and to modify their theory as necessary, seeing it as a tool and not as an end in itself.

Using models, joint education/service appointments, clinical nursing units, student-centred learning — there are many examples of good practice to be found throughout the country, often being tried out in places where there are no special resources except a great deal of determination to raise the standards of nursing care. There are also other developments which are more unconventional and politically challenging, and so receive less approval or attention from the nursing press and the nursing establishment, but which nevertheless offer very promising patterns for the future. These include community nurses organising self-help groups for people with a shared problem or need, psychiatric and mental handicap nurses living on equal terms with patients in small community homes, and nurses running well adult clinics. What these latter projects often have and what the former sometimes lack is a broader perspective to which this book is pointing — a sense of how nursing care can fit into the future needs of the community, rather than continuing in splendid, outdated and patronising isolation.

The very diversity of nursing and of nurses makes it difficult to prescribe a single way forward, and that in any case would not be a useful prescription. That diversity, and the flexibility it can encourage, is one of the chief assets which will help us to become valued and valuable practitioners of healing in the next few decades. Progress along those lines will not be easy, and it will require some very fundamental changes, not least in the way nursing sees itself and the kinds of alliances it makes. Above all it involves letting in the daylight, blowing fresh air through our stuffy corridors and taking a long, hard and honest look at who we are and at our place in the health service and society as a whole.

Further Reading

Dickson A. (1982). *A woman in your own right: assertiveness and you*. London: Quartet Books.

Hingley P. (1984). The humane face of nursing. *Nursing Mirror*; December 5, pp. 19–22.

Pearson A. (1983). *The Clinical Nursing Unit*. London: Heinemann Medical Books.

Politics of Health Group (undated). *Cuts and the NHS*. POHG pamphlet no. 2, London.

Politics of Health Group (undated). *Going private: the case against private medicine*. POHG/Fightback, London. Both available from POHG, 9 Poland Street, London W1.

Roper N., Logan W., Tierney A. (1980). *The Elements of Nursing*. Edinburgh: Churchill Livingstone.

Royal College of Nursing (1984). *Nurse Alert: a report on the effects of the financial and manpower cuts in the NHS*. London: RCN.

Ryan J. with Thomas F. (1980). *The politics of mental handicap*. Harmondsworth: Penguin Books.

Salvage J. (1983). The politics and economics of health care. In *Community Health* (Clark J., Henderson J., eds) pp. 117–26. Edinburgh: Churchill Livingstone.

Townsend P., Davidson N. (1982). *Inequalities in health: the Black report*. Harmondsworth: Penguin Books.

Appendix 1
The Statutory Bodies

The functions of the UK Central Council and the national boards include 'to maintain and improve standards of training for nurses, midwives and health visitors'.

The UK Central Council is responsible for maintaining the professional register; establishing standards of professional conduct and removing from the register the names of those guilty of serious professional misconduct; making statutory rules governing entry to training and criteria for registration; and improving standards of training, with the collaboration of the four national boards.

The national boards for England, Northern Ireland, Scotland and Wales approve institutions to provide all training/education courses for nurses, midwives and health visitors, and control examinations. They provide the direct point of contact for schools and other institutions running courses for nurses in training, or those contemplating training. They also investigate cases of alleged professional misconduct and refer serious cases to the UKCC.

Between them these five bodies have replaced and assumed the functions of the General Nursing Council for England and Wales, the GNC for Scotland, the Northern Ireland Council for Nurses and Midwives, the Central Midwives Board (England and Wales), the Central Midwives Board for Scotland, the Council for the Education and Training of Health Visitors, the Panel of Assessors for District Nurse Training, the Joint Board of Clinical Nursing Studies (England and Wales) and the Committee for Clinical Nursing Studies (Scotland).

ADDRESSES

UK Central Council for Nursing, Midwifery and Health Visiting
23 Portland Place, London W1N 3AF, tel. 01-637 7181.

The English National Board for Nursing, Midwifery and Health Visiting
Victory House, 170 Tottenham Court Road, London W1P 0HA, tel. 01-388 3131.

The National Board for Nursing, Midwifery and Health Visiting for Scotland
22 Queen Street, Edinburgh EH2 1JX, tel. 031-226 7371.

The National Board for Nursing, Midwifery and Health Visiting for Northern Ireland
RAC House, 79 Chichester Street, Belfast BT1 4JE, tel. 0232 238152.

The Welsh National Board for Nursing, Midwifery and Health Visiting
13th Floor, Pearl Assurance House, Greyfriars Road, Cardiff CF1 3RT, tel. 0222 395535.

Appendix 2
The Single Professional Register

The UKCC is required to establish a single professional register which will contain one entry for every nurse and midwife in the UK. Each entry will include every qualification that person holds. It is divided into 11 'parts' which reflect the current qualifications and titles.

TRAINING FOR ADMISSION TO PARTS 1, 3, 5 AND 8 OF THE REGISTER

These parts for the so-called 'first level nurse' incorporate the qualifications RGN/SRN, RMN, RNMS/RNMH, RSCN. Courses shall enable the student to acquire the competencies required to:

- Advise on the promotion of health and the prevention of illness.
- Recognise situations that may be detrimental to the health and well-being of the individual.
- Carry out those activities involved when conducting the comprehensive assessment of a person's nursing requirements.
- Recognise the significance of the observations made and use these to develop an initial nursing assessment.
- Devise a plan of nursing care based on the assessment with the cooperation of the patient, to the extent that this is possible, taking into account the medical prescription.
- Implement the planned programme of nursing care and where appropriate teach and coordinate other members of the caring team who may be responsible for implementing specific aspects of the nursing care.
- Review the effectiveness of the nursing care provided, and where appropriate, initiate any action that may be required.
- Work in a team with other nurses, and with medical and paramedical staff and social workers.
- Undertake the management of the care of a group of patients over a period of time and organise the appropriate support services.

The student must pass an examination held or arranged by a national board which may be in parts and is designed to assess theoretical knowledge, practical skills and attitudes, and demonstrate ability to undertake these relevant competencies.

A student who has completed training but fails on one occasion or more to pass any part of an exam testing theoretical knowledge is entitled to apply for admission to parts 2, 4, 6 or 7 of the register. These parts, for 'second level nurses', incorporate the qualifications SEN/EN, SEN(M), SEN(MS).

TRAINING FOR ADMISSION TO PARTS 2, 4, 6 AND 7 OF THE REGISTER

Courses shall provide opportunities for the student to develop the competencies required to:

- Assist in carrying out comprehensive observation of the patient and help in assessing care requirements.
- Develop skills to enable her to assist in the implementation of nursing care under the direction of a person registered in parts 1, 3, 5 or 8 of the register.
- Accept delegated nursing tasks.
- Assist in reviewing the effectiveness of the care provided.
- Work in a team with other nurses, and with medical and paramedical staff and social workers.

The student must pass an examination held or arranged by a national board which may be in parts, and which shall be designed to assess her theoretical knowledge, practical skills and attitudes and demonstrate her ability to undertake these relevant competencies.

Appendix 3
Nursing Training

TRAINING SCHOOLS

These are approved by a national board under Section 6 of the Nurses, Midwives and Health Visitors Act as training establishments providing a course of training leading to qualification for admission to a part or parts of the register.

NUMBER OF SCHOOLS

In the four UK countries around 208 institutions are approved for training registered general nurses, and 187 for general enrolled nurses. About 125 offer courses leading to registration as a psychiatric nurse (RMN) and about 90 for enrolment as a psychiatric nurse (SEN(M)). Just over 60 train registered nurses of the mentally handicapped, and 50 train enrolled nurses in the same specialty. Eight institutions train paediatric nurses (RSCN) on direct entry and nine offer a combined RSCN and general nursing course.

AGE OF ENTRY

People admitted to training must be not less than 17½ on their first day of training, or a minimum of 17 in special circumstances related to specific courses.

ENTRY REQUIREMENTS

For a registered qualification, the minimum requirements for entry to training from January 1, 1986 are five GCE O-levels (grades A, B, or C), five CSEs (grade 1), five Scottish O grades (bands A, B, or C), five Northern Ireland SCEs, five Northern Ireland GCE O-levels (grades A, B, or C), other qualifications considered to be equivalent by the UKCC, or a specified pass standard in an educational test approved by the UKCC, For enrolment the minimum requirement is evidence of having attained a good standard of general education extending over at least 10 years. These requirements are the minimum and many schools require higher standards.

THE ENTRANCE TEST

The test set by the statutory body is discretionary — i.e. schools of nursing are not obliged to offer it as an alternative to their entry requirements.

EXAMINATION SUBJECTS PREFERRED

Applicants must have O-levels (or the equivalent) in English language, English literature or history. No combination of subjects is a guarantee of acceptance but passes in the following subjects are particularly useful when applying — physics, chemistry, biology, human biology, mathematics, sociology, economics, geography, foreign languages.

WHEN TO APPLY

Schools are not usually prepared to offer a place pending exam results. Most have two or three intakes a year. Some give preference to applicants living locally. As there is as yet no central application scheme, applicants must write direct to their preferred schools, stating the course they wish to apply for, details of educational qualifications, personal details such as date of birth, and mention of any employment or voluntary work.

Attendance at a pre-nursing course does not guarantee a place at a school of nursing and academic qualifications are regarded as the greatest priority. Waiting lists vary according to specialty and location but at present they tend to be about 18 months.

GENERAL CAREERS INFORMATION

In England and Wales information on nursing careers, training and special courses such as degrees in nursing can be obtained by writing (with SAE) to the ENB Careers Advisory Centre, 26 Margaret Street, London W1N 7LB.

In Scotland, write to the Scottish Health Service Centre, Crewe Road South, Edinburgh EH4 2LF. In Northern Ireland the address is Nurse Recruitment Officer, NI National Board, 123–137 York Street, Belfast BT15 1JB.

Appendix 4
Useful Addresses

STATUTORY BODIES
See Appendix 1.

UNIONS AND PROFESSIONAL BODIES

Association of Health and Residential Care Officers (AHRCO)
c/o R. Phillips (Secretary), 11 Man Road, Cuddington, Northwich, Cheshire CW8 2XQ.

Association of Nurse Administrators (ANA)
178 High Holborn, WC1V 7AN, tel. 01-240 9784.

Association of Supervisors of Midwives (ASM)
c/o Hon. Sec. E. Guest, James Paget Hospital, Gorleston, Great Yarmouth, Norfolk, tel. 0493 600611.

Community Mental Handicap Nurses Association
28 Pendlebury Road, Swinton, Manchester M27 1AR, tel. 061794 2888.

Community Psychiatric Nurses Association
c/o Heather Rankin (Secretary), Gloucester House, Southmead Hospital, Westbury-on-Trym, Bristol BS10 5NB, tel. 0272 505050, ext. Gloucester House.

Confederation of Health Service Employees (COHSE)
Glen House, High Street, Banstead, Surrey SM7 2LH, tel. 07373 53322.

District Nursing Association
57 Lower Belgrave Street, London SW1W 0LR, or 26 Castle Terrace, Edinburgh EH1 2EL, tel. 031-229 7717.

Health Visitors Association
36 Eccleston Square, London SW1V 1PF, tel. 01-834 9523.

Managerial, Administrative, Technical and Supervisory Association (MATSA)
Thorn House, Ruxley Ridge, Claygate, Esher, Surrey KT10 0TL.

National Union of Public Employees (NUPE)
Civic House, 20 Grand Depot Road, London SE18 6SF,
tel. 01-854 2244.

Psychiatric Nurses Association
c/o A. F. Morley (President), DNS, St Nicholas' Hospital,
Gosforth, Newcastle-upon-Tyne NE3 3XT, tel. 0632 850151.

Royal College of Midwives
15 Mansfield Street, London W1M 0BE, tel. 01-580 6523.

Royal College of Nursing
20 Cavendish Square, London W1M 0AB, tel. 01-409 3333.

Scottish Association of Nurse Administrators (SANA)
c/o H. S. Bald (Hon. Sec.), Whitehills Hospital, Forsar, Angus,
Scotland DD8 3DY, tel. 0307 64551.

Scottish Health Visitors Association (SHVA)
47 Timber Bush, Leith, Edinburgh EH6 6QH, tel. 031-553 5233.

JOURNALS

Hazards
PO Box 199, Sheffield S1 1FQ.

Health Services (COHSE monthly journal)
Glen House, High Street, Banstead, Surrey SM7 2LH, tel. 07373
53322.

Health Visitor
36 Eccleston Square, London SW1V 1PF, tel. 01-834 9523.

International Journal of Nursing Studies
Pergamon Press, Headington Hill Hall, Oxford OX3 0BW.

International Nursing Review
ICN, 3 rue L'Ancien-Port, CH 1201 Geneva, Switzerland.

Journal of Advanced Nursing
Blackwell Scientific Publications Ltd, 8 John Street, London
WC1 N2ES.

Journal of District Nursing
PTM Publishers Ltd, 282 High Street, Sutton, Surrey SM1 1PQ,
tel. 01-642 0162.

Lampada
Royal College of Nursing, 20 Cavendish Square, London
W1M 0AB, tel. 01-409 2585.

Medicine in Society
16 St John Street, London EC1M 4AY.

Midwife, Health Visitor and Community Nurse
Recorder House, Stoke Newington Church Street, London
N16 0AU, tel. 01-254 7231.

Midwives Chronicle
98 Belsize Lane, London NW3 5BB, tel. 01-794 2336.

NUPE Journal
Civic House, 20 Grand Depot Road, London SE18 6SF, tel.
01-854 2244.

Nurse Education Today
Churchill Livingstone, Robert Stevenson House, 1–3 Baxter's
Place, Leith Walk, Edinburgh EH1 3AF.

Nursing (the Add-on Journal of Clinical Nursing)
Medical Education Ltd, Pembroke House, 36/37 Pembroke
Street, Oxford OX1 1BL, tel. 0865 724631.

Nursing Mirror
Surrey House, 1 Throwley Way, Sutton, Surrey SM1 4QQ, tel.
01-643 8040.

Nursing Standard
Royal College of Nursing, 20 Cavendish Square, London
W1M 0AB, tel. 01-409 2585.

Nursing Times
4 Little Essex Street, London WC2R 3LF, tel. 01-836 1776.

Radical Community Medicine
5 Lyndon Drive, Liverpool L18 6HP, tel. 051-709 9290.

INTEREST GROUPS AND RESOURCE CENTRES

Association of Radical Midwives
8A The Drive, Wimbledon, London SW20, tel. 01-504 2010.

King's Fund Centre
126 Albert Street, London NW1 7NF, tel. 01-267 6111.

Politics of Health Group
c/o BSSRS, 9 Poland Street, London W1V 3DG.

Radical Health Visitors Group
c/o BSSRS, 9 Poland Street, London W1V 3DG.

Radical Nurses Group
20 Melrose Road, Sheffield 3 and c/o BSSRS, 9 Poland Street, London W1V 3DG.

Socialist Health Association
195 Walworth Road, London SE19 1RP, tel. 01-703 6838.

Training in Health and Race
18 Victoria Park Square, London E2 9PF, tel. 01-980 6263.

Women's Health Information Centre
52 Featherstone Street, London EC1, tel. 01-251 6580.

Women's Therapy Centre
6 Manor Gardens, London N7 6LA, tel. 01-263 6200.

GOVERNMENT OFFICES AND POLITICAL PARTIES

Conservative Party
32 Smith Square, London SW1P 3HH, tel. 01-222 9000.

Department of Health and Social Security
Alexander Fleming House, Elephant and Castle, London SE1 6BY, tel. 01-407 5522.

Health and Safety Executive
25 Chapel Street, London NW1 5DT, tel. 01-262 3277.

House of Commons
Westminster, London SW1A 0AA, tel. 01-219 3000.

Labour Party
150 Walworth Road, London SE17 1JT, tel. 01-703 0833.

Liberal Party
1 Whitehall Place, London SW1A 2HE, tel. 01-839 4092.

SDP
4 Cowley Street, London SW1P 3NB, tel. 01-222 7999.

MAJOR QUANGOS

Association of Community Health Councils for England and Wales
Mark Lemon Suite, Barclays Bank Chambers, 254 Seven Sisters Road, London NW4 2HZ, tel. 01-272 5459.

Association of Scottish Local Health Councils
21 Torphichen Street, Edinburgh EH3 8HX, tel. 031-229 2344.

Association of Welsh Community Health Councils
c/o Ceredigion CHC, 5 Chalybeate Street, Aberystwyth, tel. Dyfed 4760.

Commission for Racial Equality
Elliot House, 10–12 Allington Street, London SW1E 5EH, tel. 01-828 7022.

Equal Opportunities Commission
Overseas House, Quay Street, Manchester M3 3HN, tel. 061-833 9244.

Index